I TOLD YOU I WAS ILL

I TOLD YOU I WAS ILL
Adventures in Hypochondria

John O'Connell

＊ SHORT BOOKS

First published in 2005 by
Short Books
3A Exmouth House
Pine Street
EC1R 0JH

This paperback edition published in 2006
10 9 8 7 6 5 4 3 2 1

A CIP catalogue record for this book
is available from the British Library.

ISBN   1-904977-44-8
(978-1-904977-44-5)

Printed in Great Britain by Bookmarque ltd, Croydon, Surrey

For Cathy and Scarlett

We have more nervous diseases, since the present Age has made Efforts to go beyond former Times, in all the Arts of Ingenuity, Invention, Study, Learning, and all the Contemplative and Sedentary Professions.

George Cheyne, *The English Malady* (1733)

I HAD TO DO SOMETHING

For a while now, a spot on my chest has been bothering me. It's on the right-hand side, third rib down, north-north-east of the nipple.

I say 'spot'. It used to be a spot. That's how it started – as a no-nonsense, common-or-garden whitehead. I remember it appeared suddenly, unexpectedly, without the premonitory subcutaneous lump you usually get with whiteheads. It was very swollen, very tender, more so than most whiteheads, and it hung around for weeks without showing the slightest interest in becoming less swollen or tender, or indeed in 'ripening' (my mother's phrase) into one of the Pompeiian pus volcanoes of my adolescence.

I asked my wife: 'What do you think I should do?'

'What, generally? In life?'

'About my spot.'

She made an Evelyn Waugh face. 'Leave it. You should always leave spots.'

'But it really hurts. If I put pressure on it, I get this pain sort of radiating out across my chest.'

'Then don't put pressure on it.' She turned away, back to her newspaper. 'Honestly.'

I had to do something. As I said, the spot was painful. It looked ugly, too. I'd stopped wearing shirts to work because it was visible, in the sense that an elephant is visible, with the two top buttons undone, the way I always wear shirts. I'd started wearing T-shirts every day. But all the T-shirts I owned were fitting, which is to say constricting. I wasn't going to start wearing tent-like, Christian-summer-camp T-shirts just because of some stupid spot, but all the same there was a danger with these constricting/fitting T-shirts that excessive pressure would be exerted across my ribs when I stretched or reached up to grab a hand-strap on the tube or something and the thin film of skin over the spot would rupture and...

Enough.

I filled a bowl with freshly boiled water into which I drizzled 5ml of TCP. I took a clean flannel from the laundry cupboard. I took the smallest needle I could find and sterilised it by placing it in a pan of boiling water for five minutes.

The spot was now approximately half a centimetre in diameter, with a yolky eye in the middle. The yolky eye was the locus of infection – Pus Central. Gingerly, I laid the hot flannel on it for five minutes to soften it up. Then I dug in, thinking vague thoughts about bayonets and the fake 'putrefaction' smell they pump out while you're wandering around the Trench Experience at the Imperial War Museum.

There was a brief starburst of pure pain; then all the goo came pouring out, both less and more than I expected. (I caught most of it in the flannel.)

I washed the wound and dabbed it with the flannel until it had stopped weeping. I hadn't anticipated sudden deflation. At the same time, I hadn't anticipated the swelling to double in size so that it resembled half a boiled egg implanted in my chest. Life is full of surprises.

I squirted half a tube of Savlon over the mound. I covered it in a thick wad of gauze, stuck down at the edges with proper, no-expense-spared surgical tape. And that, I thought, was that.

NOT THE WHOLE STORY

I am 33 years old. Height: just under six foot. Weight: ten and a half stone. Waist size: 32 on a good day. I have never been seriously ill or had an operation that required a general anaesthetic. I'm not allergic to anything that I know of, apart from magical realist novels, films starring Kate Beckinsale, and group holidays in rented villas.

Increasingly, though, I worry. I worry about illness and death.

I was born two months premature, an identical twin. My brother, Richard, died of respiratory failure after three days. When my parents brought me home from the hospital, my bones were still so soft that my mother had to keep turning me over in my Moses basket so that my face didn't slip out of shape. One night, she fell into a deep sleep and forgot. To this day, she maintains that my face is lop-sided. I maintain, *pace* Blake, that symmetry is fearful.

None of this augured well. But look! – here I am, against the odds.

Do I live healthily? Kind of. But this healthy living is passive rather than active. It consists of not doing things (eating junk food, smoking, drinking to excess) rather than doing them (exercising). And apparently this is not good enough, not any more, not at my age.

'You never exercise,' says my wife, who does exercise, three times a week. She hires a personal trainer, a wiry tri-athlete called Helen.

Helen comes to our house in the morning, early. When she knocks I shuffle to the door in my dressing gown, coffee in hand. Then I call upstairs: 'Whippet woman's here!'

'Don't call her that.'

'What? Who?'

'Helen. Don't call her whippet woman.'

'Why not?'

'It isn't nice.'

I let Helen in. 'Hello,' says Helen, all smiles. 'How are you?'

Cathy skips down the stairs, dressed for action. She tells Helen, 'He's worrying about his health again.'

Helen turns towards me. 'It was your prostate, wasn't it?'

Cathy rolls her eyes. 'Last month, yeah.'

Helen, a sensible woman, has no wish to get caught up in some tedious marital micro-spat; but in the end her urge to be polite gets the better of her. 'What's the worry now?'

Cathy answers before I can. 'He had a spot on his chest. But he popped it and it went septic. Now it won't heal.'

This is factually accurate. But it isn't the whole story. The whole story... Well, that's a different matter. The whole story of my spot is a passable introduction to a bigger story whose erratic, tachycardiac rhythms compel more of us than we might care to admit: the story of hypochondria.

A DISEASE IN ITSELF

Over the past few thousand years, the word 'hypochondria' has accrued more meanings than a plague victim has weeping buboes. (Black death is on its way back, by the way.) But let's start with the most common: the contemporary meaning – the definition that springs most readily to mind when you hear the word. According to the American Psychiatric Association's *Diagnostic and Statistical Manual of Mental Disorders, 4th Edition* (DSM-IV, 1994), it's a preoccupation with the fear or idea of having a serious illness, based upon a misinterpretation of bodily sensations. This fear or idea must persist for at least six months despite appropriate medical examination and reassurance.

The Royal College of General Practitioners in the UK estimates that 25 per cent of all consultations with GPs relate to psychosomatic or unexplained symptoms. According to US figures, over $20 billion a year is spent keeping hypochondriacs happy with unnecessary medical treatments.

At its most extreme, then, hypochondria is a medical condition in its own right, a disease in itself which needs, as the jargon has it, to be 'positively diagnosed'. This means it's not enough to rule out physical disease in a patient. The grounds for his conviction that he is ill must also be established.

Its manifestations can be extreme. Writer Carla Cantor found herself locked up in the psychiatric ward of her local hospital after she became convinced she had the autoimmune disease lupus. 'Each day during the winter of 1983, I'd catalogue my lupus-like symptoms – joint aches, rashes, itching attacks, black and blue marks, exhaustion. I'd bring the list to the doctors, begging them to confirm my diagnosis,' she writes in *Phantom Illness*, the book about her condition she co-authored with psychologist Brian Fallon. On that occasion her doctors managed to convince her that there was nothing physically wrong; but the symptoms' recurrence ten years later she saw as confirmation of her initial suspicions. 'Tests were negative, but no matter how many doctors tried to reassure me that I didn't have lupus I wasn't convinced. I knew about the bizarre and fluctuating symptoms that make lupus so tough to diagnose and that no test was entirely accurate in ruling it out.'

Eventually Cantor accepted her doctors' diagnosis: clinical depression. Fallon, whom she turned to for treatment, prescribed Prozac – this was the early 1990s, and he was researching the effects of those then new 'wonder drugs', selective serotonin reuptake inhibitors (SSRIs), on hypochondria. Fallon scored a success, and within months Cantor's life was handed back to her, mended.

Paul Salkovskis, clinical director of the Centre for Anxiety Disorders at London's Maudsley hospital, doesn't even use the term 'hypochondria'. He prefers 'persistent health anxiety'. 'People get anxious about what is important to them,' he told the *Guardian* (March 4, 2001), 'and of course health is very important to most people. Those with severe health anxiety seem to interpret their bodily variations differently from other people, though. This may not just come from physical sensation but also from something heard on the radio, read in a magazine or seen on television. For those with severe health anxiety, the information will trigger feelings of hyper-awareness of the body which are very real and need to be taken very seriously.'

This, then, is the modern way – kindly, tolerant, empathetic. But all too often the old stereotype prevails. A manual dating from 1914, *The Modern Family Doctor*, attributes hypochondria to insufficient backbone – to moral weakness and cowardice.

Hypochondriacs, says the book, 'remain childlike, egoistic and self-centred, and they may be specious, plausible and good at making excuses'. They have 'no kindliness of heart, no love of country':

'Advice is generally futile to the hypochondriac. It is like trying to whistle down the wind, for no sooner do you succeed in getting one false idea out of his head than another replaces it. There is an Italian proverb that runs: "He who scrubs the head of an ass wastes his own soap."'

The problem is, most hypochondriacs aren't serious hypochondriacs. They're people like me, mid-spectrum hypochondriacs – concerned about their health to the point where their friends and colleagues laugh at them, but not to the point where they need actual treatment. Mid-spectrum hypochondriacs think their hypochondria is essentially sensible, and that their concerns are intelligent and rational. Their reaction to

Brian Fallon's definition of the condition as an 'excessive focus on benign symptoms' would be: Benign to whom?

IN A SPIN

This is the tricky bit. When does rational concern about a symptom or group of symptoms spill over into irrational obsession?

At 66, three times Formula One world champion Sir Jackie Stewart remains a busy man, with a mass of consultancies and presidencies and trusteeships. He's a professional risk-taker – not many people's idea of a hypochondriac. Yet every year for the past 20 years, Sir Jackie has flown his wife and two sons to the Mayo Clinic in Minnesota for in-depth health checks in which every inch of their bodies is scanned. In March 2000, thanks to these tests, Sir Jackie's eldest son, Paul, was found to have a potentially fatal type of cancer – non-Hodgkin's lymphoma of the colon. A few months later his wife, Helen, was diagnosed with breast cancer. Finally, to set the seal on his *annus horribilis*, Sir Jackie himself was found to have a malignant melanoma on his right cheek.

17

In an interview with the *Financial Times* (November 29, 2003), Sir Jackie admitted that he was 'put in a spin' by this cancer triple-whammy: 'Luckily I had the best connections in the world in terms of the medical aid required. I've a lot of sympathy for people who may not be as fortunate as me in having access to resources.'

It's more than just a question of resources, though. Vigilance like his is a function of a particular mindset, one most doctors would dismiss as hypochondriacal. Sir Jackie, these doctors would say, is a 'somatiser' – excessively preoccupied with the state of his body.

Is this a good thing or a bad thing?

FEAR AND ANXIETY

Psychoanalysts like to distinguish between 'fear' and 'anxiety'. They invoke the case of Little Hans, a boy of five who was treated by his father under Freud's supervision. Little Hans was so frightened of being bitten by a horse in the street that he refused to go outside. 'Hans's anxiety,' writes Freud, 'which thus corresponded to a repressed erotic longing, was, like every infantile anxiety, without an object to begin with; it was still anxiety not yet fear.' In other words, fear is focused on a specific, real object or situation; anxiety is detached from its object – generalised, abstract, irrational.

(Hans's father told Freud that his son's problem 'seems somehow connected with his having been frightened by a large penis'. But that's another story.)

Is hypochondria a fear or an anxiety? It depends, I guess, on how 'specific' and 'real' your specific, real object or situation is.

BODY OR WAFER?

It is 1981. I am nine years old and at Sunday school, which happens after mass. Mass is really boring. My mother says it was more interesting when it was in Latin but then something called Vatican II happened which sounds like a space ship but was actually a ruling by the Pope who was shot but didn't die. She says that now mass is in English it has 'lost all its mystery'.

Today we are learning about why bodies are important if you are a Catholic. They are important because you need one to get to Heaven. If you get cremated then you can't go to Heaven because you won't be whole, so you won't rise on Judgement Day. So your body needs to be intact, which means not in pieces or damaged.

This is what Father Dillon says. But then, Father Dillon says lots of things. He says that the communion wafer isn't just a wafer – it's Jesus's body. He makes us write down a word – TRANSUBSTANTIATION. It's the longest word I've ever heard. It's the word for what happens when a wafer becomes a body, which doesn't make sense because how can a wafer become a body any more than a car can become a tree? Still, it makes sense to Father Dillon, and he's a grown-up, so he must know what he's talking about.

Also, he's a priest, so he has faith, which we learned about last week. Faith means believing in things when they're not there. Very holy people are born with it. Everyone else must work hard to acquire it.

Father Dillon tells us a story about a town that was evacuated during a flood. A group of children ran to the church because they realised that Jesus was alone in the tabernacle and they needed to save Him and keep Him company. They realised He was a person, not just a wafer.

Roger, who has red hair and smells, asks: 'What if you sick up after communion? Can you wipe it up or do you have to eat it again because it's Jesus and you can't just leave Him on the floor?'

'That's a very good question,' says Father Dillon twinklingly, 'and you're not going to like the answer. Because the answer is… yes!'

Father Dillon likes to make an impression. He reads to us from a magazine called the *Junior Catholic Messenger*. Today he is reading an article about how, when we're in church, we should always be thinking about our bodies and what we're doing with them – how we kneel and bow and genuflect.

Look at the crucifix – at the damage Jesus's body sustained on our behalf! The least we can do is receive communion properly – eyes cast down, hands pressed together so that the palms touch.

Later, at home, my mother asks, 'How was Sunday school?'

I tell her: 'Father Dillon said we should eat our own sick.'

Next week, we go straight home after mass and have lunch early, which is good.

A PLATONIC IDEAL OF WELLNESS

For doctors, one of the most frustrating things about hypochondriacs is their belief that it's possible to feel completely well all the time. This leads them, they say, to interpret any physical symptom as a sign that something is wrong.

> **Indoor air pollution is responsible for 2.7 per cent of the global burden of disease.**

But does it? Unless you've always suffered from some sort of chronic condition, surely it is possible to feel completely well, or at least to know what it is to feel well (based on a memory of childhood, perhaps, or the immediate aftermath of a corrective operation). I think most people carry around with them a Platonic ideal of wellness.

They know when they are well – when their bodies and minds are in a state of benign equilibrium – and when they are not.

The test which psychologists use to diagnose hypochondria is called the Whitely Index. It comprises 14 questions, answers to which are graded from 1 to 5 in rising order of severity. It's an interesting test to try out on yourself. (My own answers are beneath the questions in italics.)

The Whitely Index

1. Do you worry about your health?
Yes, obviously. (5)

2. Do you think there is something seriously wrong with your body?
Not seriously wrong – not at the moment. (2)

3. Is it hard for you to forget about yourself and think about all sorts of other things?
It depends on how bad a headache I have at the time. (3)

4. If you feel ill and someone tells you that you are looking better, do you become annoyed?
It depends how they say it, whether I think they're

being sarcastic, etc. If it's an obvious lie – if I'm feeling
ill and know for certain that I look terrible – of course
I'll become annoyed. (3)

5. Do you find that you are often aware of various things happening in your body?
Yes. (This is really a question about poo, isn't it?) (5)

6. Are you bothered by many aches and pains?
How many is 'many'? Five? Six? I'd say I'm bothered by 'some'. (3)

7. Are you afraid of illness?
Of course. (5)

8. Do you worry about your health more than most people?
I think most people worry about their health quite a lot, so no. (1)

9. Do you get the feeling that people are not taking your illnesses seriously enough?
Almost always. (5)

10. Is it hard for you to believe the doctor when he/she

tells you there is nothing for you to worry about?
Yes. (5)

11. Do you often worry about the possibility that you have a serious illness?
Yes. (5)

12. If a disease is brought to your attention (through the radio, TV, newspapers or someone you know), do you worry about getting it yourself?
Yes. (5)

13. Do you find that you are bothered by many different symptoms?
See answer to 6. (3)

14. Do you often have the symptoms of a very serious disease?
Stupid question. Everyone knows that lots of very serious diseases are symptomless in their early stages. (3)

Healthy people without health anxiety generally have a score of 21 +/-7 (14-28). Patients with hypochondria generally have a score of 44 +/-11 (32 to 55).

My score is 53. I guess this makes me a hypochondriac. But

this is absurd, surely? Any reasonably intelligent person would score over 44 on this test, wouldn't they?

Wouldn't they?

HE TOLD US HE WAS ILL

Asked what he would like as his epitaph, the writer and come-dian Spike Milligan replied, 'I told you I was ill.'

It's a good joke because of what it reveals about the hypochondriac mindset. For the hypochondriac, vindication is all-important. For the hypochondriac, life is one long episode of *The Prisoner*. You are Number 6, trapped in your own private Portmeirion of symptomatic abundance, while all around you conspiracy rages – a conspiracy of denial and slander and obfuscation.

No wonder hypochondriacs get cross. And no wonder most doctors hate them. There are lots of derogatory names for hypochondriacs. The most euphemistic is 'the worried well', which packs a harder punch than its poetic mien implies, though it's still preferable to the medical slang terms – 'crock', 'turkey', 'GOMER' (it stands for Get Out of My Emergency Room) and 'heartsink patients'.

I tell myself I can't be a proper, in-need-of-treatment hypochondriac because they go to see their doctors every week and I only go once a month, or thereabouts.

But I'm deluding myself here. I'm not counting the additional visits I make to the private drop-in clinics which have opened across London over the last few years. Medicentres, they're called. There's one at Victoria Station and another on Oxford Street – perfect, convenient locations if you work in central London. The doctors are all South African, and they don't let your NHS doctor know anything about your visit unless you want them to. It's expensive – £55 per consultation – but worth it for peace of mind. And they're so polite and tolerant and interested!

'Of course they are,' says Cathy. 'You're paying them to be.'

I concede that this is true.

CHOLESTEROL

It's just before Christmas, 1983. I am 11 years old, and living with my mother and sister in Market Drayton, a small town on the border of Shropshire and Staffordshire. If I'm honest, our house isn't really in Market Drayton, it's four miles to the north in a village called, on account of its position at a crossroads, Loggerheads. But we have learned the hard way not to say 'At Loggerheads' when people ask us where we live.

Market Drayton's only real draw is a big supermarket called Fine Fare, now extinct. Fine Fare has a garish, electric-orange logo which seems to seep into the décor and the food. We go

26

shopping there on Saturdays – or rather, my mother goes shopping while my sister and I skulk around Woolworths.

(Alex has recently discovered that you can fit up to three seven-inch singles in the sleeve of a 12-inch single without the person on the till noticing. I'm far too scared to attempt anything like this. Which is pathetic, really – especially as Alex is 18 months younger than me.

'You worry too much,' Alex tells me.

'What about?' I ask.

'Everything.'

She's right.)

Every Saturday, as a special treat, our mother buys us each a vanilla millefeuille slice. When you bite into it, the = gloopy-sweet, fridge-cold filling oozes out at the sides and makes, if you're not careful, a right mess. The slices come in a cardboard box with a flip-up lid. Sometimes, if we're really hungry, we eat them in the car on the way home, but we always regret this later: they taste much better with the bitter, espresso-strength coffee we have been raised to consume by the mugful.

Today, however, I don't want my vanilla slice. In fact, I'm looking at it in a whole new light. Where once I saw crisp puff pastry and golden confectioners' custard, now I see only cholesterol.

I have recently become rather obsessed with cholesterol. The other night I watched a *Horizon* documentary about what happened to the arteries in your heart when you ate too much fatty food. Normally I try to avoid watching *Horizon* in front of my mother and sister in case there's something about human reproduction in it (there often is – you never can tell), but this one was so gripping I forgot to care. A man who was nearly dead from heart disease had allowed the BBC to put a camera right inside his heart! You could see all the cholesterol really clearly. It was like a fungus growing on the walls of his arteries. In some places it was so thick that the blood couldn't get through. The programme explained that when this happened, you had a heart attack and almost always died.

How will you die? Rate your chances...

Complications of hospital care: 1 in 1,170
Riding a motorbike: 1 in 1,295
Fatal air accident: 1 in 4,608
Being accidentally shot: 1 in 4,613
Tripping over on level ground: 1 in 6,336
Falling off a ladder: 1 in 8,689
Choking on your own vomit: 1 in 9,372
Driving in a heavy truck: 1 in 9, 702
Drowning in the bath: 1 in 10,948
Suffocating in bed: 1 in 10,948
Scalded by hot tap water: 1 in 65, 092
Hornet, wasp or bee stings: 1 in 66,297
In a three-wheeled vehicle: 1 in 155,654
On foot: 1 in 610
Fireworks: 1 in 716,010
Venomous spiders: 1 in 716,010

Source:
American National Safety Council's
Lifetime Risk of Death Study **(2000)**

It's tricky, knowing this, to look at a vanilla millefeuille slice and not see Death.

Since the programme, nothing has been able to distract me from The Certainty of Death By Heart Attack – not even the knowledge that experts have developed a new technique called angioplasty which involves inflating a balloon (a balloon!) inside the arteries, thereby dispersing the cholesterol. A demonstration of this technique was actually the crux of the *Horizon* in question, but for some reason this hasn't reassured me.

With immediate effect, I cut out (as far as I am able: it's not like I actually cook or anything) cream and eggs from my diet. Fat I leave behind on my plate. I start eating foul, pellety Bran Buds for breakfast, and shake my head when I am offered what was previously my favourite pudding ever – two Mr Kipling apple pies heated in the microwave so that the pastry softens, served with two scoops of Wall's Golden Vanilla ice cream.

Christmas Day arrives, and with it a book called *The Pears Encyclopedia of Child Health*. This is a present from my mother. It is by Drs Andrew and Penny Stanway, unbelievably prolific medical writers who will, in the early 1990s, acquire mild notoriety for their involvement in a self-help video called *The Lovers' Guide* which showed a couple *actually having sex*.

Its purpose is clearly twofold. It is supposed to help me

learn all I can about diseases (with specific reference to cardiopulmonary failure). But it is also meant to supply much-needed perspective – to say, effectively:

Here are some things that might go wrong with you. Some of them might kill you, but realistically most of them won't. And anyway, since you're so interested in this stuff, why not work a bit harder at school and become a doctor like your grandfather? Then you can have the inscribed barometer he was awarded when he retired. He was also called John O'Connell, so for you to follow in his footsteps would be good and neat and rightful, wouldn't it?

Think about it, anyway.

No pressure.

Within hours, the encyclopedia has become my new favourite book, displacing Roald Dahl's *Tales of the Unexpected* and *Fluke* by James Herbert.

The first entry is 'abdomen', which the Stanways define as 'the part of the body between the diaphragm and the pelvis'. (Fine, but what's a diaphragm when it's at home?)

The last entry is 'worms'. 'Several different sorts of worms can live in the human body,' reveal the Stanways, 'and though many are commoner in tropical countries, they occur worldwide.'

There are pictures. A boy with measles, his face a colander of tiny red spots. An obese boy, naked, with rickety legs and a black stripe across his eyes, standing next to a height chart. A breastfeeding woman, her chestnut nipples plainly and – to my puritanical, prepubescent mind – obscenely visible. (Over the coming years I will return to this page with a more tolerant, even easygoing attitude towards breasts.)

I look up 'cholesterol', but there isn't an entry for it – a gross oversight on the Stanways' part. Don't they know that within 20 years cholesterol will have KILLED US ALL? I write to them via their publisher – the third 'fan' letter I have written (the others were to Roald Dahl and Kate Bush), but the first, admittedly, to strike a vaguely reproving tone.

I never receive a reply.

***

From this moment on, hypochondria gatecrashes my life. Thousands of tiny health-related worries appear out of nowhere and assume elephantine proportions. I can no longer allow myself to drink coffee in case I suffer a caffeine-related heart attack; stroke Pickles, our cat, in case I contract toxoplasmosis; or eat white bread lest the fibrelessness of my diet trigger the condition that scares me the most – a prolapse of the rectum.

Again and again, my eyes scan the encyclopedia entry.

Prolapse.

Rectum.

Prolapse.

Rectum.

Prolapserectumprolapserectum.

It can't happen, can it? It's too hideous even to contemplate. And how loftily unfazed the Stanways are!

'Treatment is simple,' they declare. 'Lie the child down and raise the end of the bed on blocks or books. To push the rectum back in, wrap your finger in some tissue, insert it into the centre of the prolapse and push it back in.'

Eurrrrrrgghhhhhhhhhhhhhhhhhhhhhh!

'If you do this without paper, your finger will pull the rectum right back out again as you withdraw it.'

Aaaaaaaaaaaaaaaaaaaaarrrrrrrrghhhhhhhhhhhhhhhhhhhhhhh!

Is it anally retentive to worry about your bottom falling out?

***

The author of *The Modern Family Doctor* would have thought me a disgrace; for although he's surprisingly indulgent of 'nervous children' – 'It is from this class that the infant prodigies and geniuses arise' – his sympathy has vanished by the time he gets round to considering adolescence:

'With the arrival of full manhood should come altruism – that quality upon which organised society is built,' he observes. 'Did we all remain egoistic boys and girls, society, as we understand it, would be impossible. Martial gave us long ago the note of the sane and healthy man: "To look on death with placid eye,/And neither fear nor wish to die." With the neurasthenic and hypochondriac it is quite otherwise.'

A VISIT TO GIMPFACE

The spot on my chest is now a shiny red weal, the skin around it flaky and itchy and eczematous. I've started putting hydrocortisone cream on it, but I have to be careful not to get any on the weal itself. Hydrocortisone cream thins the skin over time, and the skin covering the weal is already like gossamer. When I towel myself after a bath, it comes off. When my shirt rubs against it, it comes off. The result is profuse bleeding which can take up to fifteen minutes to stop. Sometimes the only way I can make it stop is to hold a pack of frozen peas against it. Afterwards I cover it with a plaster, which works fine in the short term, but often I'll nick the skin in the process of removing the plaster and the bleeding will start all over again.

This goes on for several weeks. I would like it to be known that only after it had been going on for several weeks did I decide to visit my GP.

I tell Cathy: 'I'm going to Gimpface tomorrow.'

'About your spot?' She sounds only mildly incredulous.

'Yeah.'

'Well,' she says, 'if it makes you feel better.'

***

Gimpface is our name for our GP. I cannot, in all honesty, pretend that this is a friendly nickname. On the contrary, it is a nickname conceived in fury after he misdiagnosed Cathy's shingles as ringworm a couple of years back.

The surgery is about ten minutes walk away. I decide to take a detour past our local garage. It's a Shell garage, adjacent to one of the many ornate Victorian railway bridges you find around our bit of south London. The other day, we received a hand-delivered letter informing us that Hutchison 3G, the mobile phone company, was intending to erect a mast to the rear of the forecourt. The letter was not from Hutchison 3G or Southwark Council. It was from local campaigners against the mast.

I have read about the perceived risks of mobile phone masts – of cancer clusters, rashes, nausea, dizziness, nosebleeds. I don't know whether to believe the campaigners or the authorities. I want to believe the authorities. It's easier that way. I want to believe the government-commissioned Stewart report into the safety of mobile phone technology, which concluded:

34

'The balance of evidence does not suggest that mobile phone technologies put the health of the general population... at risk. There is some preliminary evidence that outputs from mobile phone technologies may cause, in some cases, subtle biological effects, although importantly these do not necessarily mean that health is affected.'

(What's a 'subtle biological effect'?)

For a good minute I stand in front of the garage, lips pursed, frowning, gripped by... anxiety, or fear?

Cancer cluster. It's hard to think of a more horrible phrase. Somewhere, probably in Portsmouth, there must be a crap indie band called Cancer Cluster.

Obviously, my main concern is that the spot

> **Top Ten most fatal cancers in the UK in 2002:**
>
> 1. **Lung**
> 2. **Bowel**
> 3. **Breast**
> 4. **Prostate**
> 5. **Oesophagus**
> 6. **Pancreas**
> 7. **Stomach**
> 8. **Bladder**
> 9. **Non-Hodgkin's lymphoma**
> 10. **Ovary**
>
> **Source: Cancer Research**

on my chest is cancerous. That's why I'm so keen for the doctor to see it. We're always being encouraged to alert our doctors to funny-looking, itchy moles and that sort of thing. My spot falls into the 'that sort of thing' category. It's definitely not a mole, but it did just appear suddenly out of nowhere. It bleeds and itches. And bleeding and itching is bad, isn't it?

The waiting room is packed. Opposite me sits one of the fattest women I have ever seen. Her thighs ooze out and under the narrow wooden chair like melting marshmallow. Febrile toddlers run amok; you can almost see the steam coming off them. Their mothers call after them feebly: 'John-Luke! JOHN-LUKE! Get over here – now!'

It's a funny old surgery. (We've since switched.) Doctors have a habit of leaving, and when they do it's as if either the ground has swallowed them or they never existed in the first place. When I was queuing at the reception desk, the old woman in front of me asked if she'd be seeing Dr Redmond, the doctor she liked best.

'Oh no,' said the receptionist. 'He doesn't work here any more.'

'He did two weeks ago,' reasoned the old lady.

'Well, that was two weeks ago.'

'I know. That's what I said.'

'A lot can happen in two weeks.'

'Not that much,' said the old lady, sadly. 'Not when you get to my age.'

On the table in front of me is a pile of magazines. Old, torn magazines, much thumbed. Most of them are women's mags, their covers aglow with soap stars I don't recognise. None of them appeals much. My attention is caught, however, by a copy of *Reader's Digest* (September 2004 issue). The coverline is: 'Need A Laugh? 50 Best Jokes Ever!'

Vacantly, I flick through the issue in search of the best jokes ever. But I never find them. I am distracted en route by the story of David Perkins from Collingham in West Yorkshire.

'I was working on an electrical connection,' David has written in a letter to the magazine, 'when I momentarily felt an odd sensation deep in my abdomen. I thought no more about it. Then my copy of *Reader's Digest* arrived. I flicked through it and started reading "10 Diseases Doctors Miss". I read about hepatitis C, lupus, then came aneurysm. Lo and behold, one symptom was a pulse in the stomach. I went straight to my GP. From that moment, events happened at lightning speed and I was operated on immediately, such was the danger.'

Wow, I think. An 'odd sensation' in the stomach. I have those.

David's story is on page 14. A little further along, on page 23, is the story of Olivia Giles. She left work early one day feeling shivery and thirsty. Her boyfriend called a doctor who told her she had a virus and should take an aspirin. Doh! She had meningococcal septicaemia, 'one of the most lethal forms of meningitis'! As her lungs and kidneys failed, gangrene started to gnaw away at her arms and feet. 'Robin and her family faced a ghastly choice – turn off her life-support machine or agree to amputation above her elbows and knees.'

Gosh, I think. Death versus amputation. What would I choose?

I read on. Every other article is about someone narrowly avoiding dying from a terrible, often freakishly rare disease. There's six-year-old Paris, who has xeroderma pigmentosum, 'a rare genetic condition that prevents sun-damaged skin cells from repairing themselves'. Or what about 52-year-old Jim? He had a symptomless kidney condition which would have killed him had his wife not donated him one of her kidneys.

Hmm, I think. Would Cathy donate me one of her kidneys in a similar situation? I must ask her when she gets back from work.

What is this magazine doing in a doctor's surgery?

After what feels like seven hours but is actually one hour and 12 minutes, the receptionist calls my name.

I knock on the door and Gimpface calls, 'Come in!' But when I go in, he's on the phone. It sounds like he's on the phone to his partner.

'Really?' he's saying. 'Did he say that? And what did you say?'

I cough into my hand. Gimpface ignores me.

After about five minutes (consultations are supposed to last for fifteen), Gimpface puts the phone down. 'Sorry,' he says. 'I didn't mean to press the buzzer when I did.'

'Oh.'

'They sent you in too early.'

'Right.'

Gimpface has the build and demeanour of a rugby second-row – thick neck, meaty hands, thighs that rub together when he walks. His hair looks like the hair in the Grecian 2000 adverts: subtly aerated, parting like a Roman road. His mouth is fixed in a half-smile, and his eyes twinkle merrily, as if my presence here is the most tremendous joke – as if my predicament, whatever it turns out to be, is simply grist to the hulking, steam-powered mill of his ironic sensibility.

'So,' he says. 'What seems to be the problem?'

As efficiently as I can, I explain about the spot. I try to keep the story straight – not to embellish or waffle, which I know doctors hate, with good reason. While I'm talking he stares at me, stroking his lips with his thumb.

When I've finished, he sighs and says, 'I suppose I should take a look at it then.'

I take my shirt off. He doesn't bother to get up from his chair. I say, 'It might be easier if you stood up.'

He says, 'I'm fine sitting here.'

He leans forward and peers squintingly at the spot. Then he sits back, as if stunned into silence.

Time passes.

'So?' I say.

'It's not cancer,' he says.

'I didn't ask you if it was.'

'To be absolutely honest,' he says, 'I don't know what it is.'

'Okay.'

'It looks a bit like a blood blister.'

'That's what I thought. But blood blisters go in a couple of weeks.'

'Whatever it is,' says Gimpface, 'it's so... *minor*. If you hold on a moment I'll look it up.'

From a small bookshelf just behind his desk he plucks a fat manual. He leafs through it listlessly. 'No,' he says, 'nothing here.'

'Nothing at all?'

'No.'

'And you really think it's nothing serious?'

'As I said, I don't know what it is. We could have a bash at freezing it off if you like.'

SETTING LIMITS

How should doctors deal with hypochondriacs? In the September 2003 issue of *Current Psychiatry*, Brian Fallon and Suzanne B Feinstein offer some advice. Doctors need, they say, to set limits to their involvement with 'problem patients'. They suggest doctors tell their patients something like this: 'I will reassure you only at office visits (not by phone), the office visits will be limited to once a month, and during each visit I will reassure you no more than once.'

So what I want to know is, where's my reassurance? After all, it's pretty obvious Gimpface thinks I'm a 'problem patient'.

'So,' he says, watching me put my shirt on. 'How's the old prostate?'

'I still have to get up in the night. Several times.'

'Maybe you should drink less before you go to bed.'

'I don't want you to tell me that I've got prostate cancer,' I say. 'I want you to suggest other things that might be wrong.'

But Gimpface has already pressed the buzzer.

INEQUALITIES OF KNOWLEDGE

In his book *Hippocratic Oaths: Medicine and its Discontents*, philosopher-consultant Professor Raymond Tallis laments the questioning of doctors' status in society. He complains that, where they used to be god-like, now 'they are more closely regulated than ever before'.

What really gets Professor Tallis's goat is the way that 'the idealisation of the patient as the marginalised, put-upon, disempowered victim of medicine, or of an NHS that "seems to work for its own convenience, not the patient's", ignores

41

the fact that the patient is primarily self-interested, and how his or her self-interest is potentially in conflict with that of other patients.'

Patients have, he believes, ceased to respect doctors' expertise to the point where it is becoming 'difficult for doctors to hold on to the fundamental values of compassion and empathy'. He goes on: 'The contribution of the internet to empowering patients, by abolishing the inequality of knowledge between doctor and patient, has been greatly exaggerated... An "e-hypochondriac" is no more sophisticated than one nourished on glossy magazines.'

> The seeds of cherries, plums, peaches, apricots and other fruits in the rose family contain substances called cyanogenetic glycosides which, when eaten and broken down by enzymes, release hydrogen cyanide gas. Bitter almonds are especially rich in glycosides: 8 to 10 of them can kill a child.

I'm glad Professor Tallis mentions the internet. (We will consider its empowering effect and what's become known as 'cyberchondria' a little later on.) Reasoning – incorrectly, as it happened – that Googling 'red spot that bleeds' wasn't likely to get me very far, I'd made a point of abstaining, in this instance, from my usual practice of frantic internet self-diagnosis. Besides, I do genuinely believe, in spite of how I'm sounding, that it's much better to get your symptoms appraised first-hand by a qualified professional.

But I'm so pissed off with Gimpface that I go straight online the second I get home.

Within half an hour, I have a reasonable idea of what the spot is. It's a vascular lesion – an example of what's known as telangiectasias. They're often associated with excessive sun exposure or alcohol use, but in my case it's probably down to age and congenital predisposition. When, subsequently, I tell my mother about the spot, she pulls up her sleeve and shows me scores of similar ones scattered across her arm.

'Though most are asymptomatic,' explains the *Medline Plus Medical Encyclopaedia*, 'some telangiectasias bleed readily and cause significant problems.'

Scarily, 'telangiectasias may also occur in the brain'. When they do, your number is most probably up. But such a subtle biological effect need not detain us here.

FEATHERS OF A BIRD

'Feathers from China could bring avian flu to Britain, despite the ban on poultry meat imports from that country, a micro-biologist, Professor Hugh Pennington, told BBC Radio's *Farming Today*. He said there was a real risk of the virus arriving in faecal traces on feathers being imported for purposes such as making pillows.'

Sunday Telegraph, March 6, 2005

ATHENS, IN AUGUST

The hotel receptionist paused before handing us the room key. She noticed me noticing and turned away, blushing.

Now I know what she was doing, what that pause was for. She was asking herself: Can I get away with giving them this room? Then answering, a heartbeat later: Yeah, why not?

Cathy and I stand in the doorway, taking in the view.

I say: 'We can't stay here.'

'There aren't any other rooms,' says Cathy.

'Then we should find another hotel.'

From directly outside the single window comes the crackly roar of three motorbikes surging past. Too fat to manage much in the way of reaction, the pigeons on the ledge flutter briefly before realising it's a false alarm. There are pigeon feathers all over the floor and, on the far wall, a grey-white streak of pigeon shit.

Cathy shrugs off her rucksack. 'It's Athens. In August. After a freak storm. All the decent hotels are full.'

I look around, at the narrow iron beds with their stained counterpanes; at the mat which looks and – yes – feels damply encrusted with sand shaken from the sandals of other travellers

44

who, like us, have had an unexpected night to kill here before setting out to or returning from the islands. It's obviously the hotel's emergency room, for use only when bad weather has scuppered the Piraeus ferries and people are too desperate to reject it on health-and-safety grounds.

Considered in those terms, maybe it's okay. It's somewhere to sleep. Somewhere to wash.

Somewhere to wash.

I ask Cathy: 'Didn't they say there was a bathroom?'

'Yeah. Down the corridor.'

We burst open the bathroom door like cops raiding a crack den. It's common in Greece for there to be no shower tray (so that the water runs away through a small plug-hole set in the middle of the floor), and for the room to be so small that the toilet obtrudes helplessly into what we might call the 'showering space'. It's also common for there to be no toilet seat, for the fittings to be ancient (30 years is the norm), and for there to be an overpowering smell of drains. Not any old drains either – drains down which a family of rats fed exclusively on garlic and cheese has contrived to get stuck and die.

This bathroom has all the classic attributes. But it also has an extra special something tipping it over the thin line between tolerable and disgusting: a dead pigeon, floating in the toilet bowl.

'One for the collection,' says Cathy.

Nodding in agreement, I run back to the room to fetch my camera.

A THROBBING PAIN

Bathrooms have a special place in the hypochondriac's demonology. Depressive *Carry On* actor Kenneth Williams never invited anyone back to his tiny Marylebone flat in case they asked to use the bathroom. He wrote in his diary: 'I can't stand the idea of another bottom on my loo.'

Russell Davies, who edited Williams's diaries for publication, thinks his hypochondria was exacerbated by an unusually low pain threshold. Which may be the case, but I defy you to be stoical in the face of a suppurating rectal ulcer. Williams's diary entry for March 30, 1975 ponders the ailment with characteristic frankness: 'There is a throbbing pain coming from the rectum. I've had it before but it's never lasted as long as this. The pain from the bum makes me think of death and I immediately see myself taking the overdose and imagine what my last acts would be.'

THE TOILET AEROSOL EFFECT

You don't need a degree in environmental microbiology to know that bathrooms are bacterial hot zones – though in some ways it would help if you had one. Then, you'd know all about the definitive study of the 'toilet aerosol effect', published in 1975 by Professor Charles Gerba of the University of Arizona.

Using a system of precisely positioned gauze pads, Gerba demonstrated that, after a toilet has been flushed, an invisible mist of microbes floats up to eight feet from the bowl for at least two hours. This mist typically contains streptococcus, staphylococcus, E.coli and shigella bacteria and the viruses responsible for hepatitis A and the common cold. It has a favourite target: the moist, exposed bristles of your toothbrush.

Bathrooms spread disease. Legionnaires' disease, so called because its first victims were American Legionnaires attending a convention in Philadelphia in 1976, loves whirlpool baths. The 2003 outbreak of severe acute respiratory syndrome (SARS) in the Amoy Gardens apartment complex in Hong Kong – 324 cases! – was caused by water droplets containing the SARS virus being sucked out of bathrooms by extractor fans, contaminating the building's ventilation system.

The Hong Kong SARS epidemic was traced back to a single source: a man from the Guangdong province of mainland China who had stayed at the block while visiting his brother. How had he contracted the disease? Doctors were stumped – until they discovered a virus 99 per cent similar to SARS in an animal called a palm civet, a cat-like mammal related to the mongoose whose perineal glands yield a musky substance used in many Western perfumes. Palm civets are indigenous to the Guangdong province where (drum roll, please) they are bred and slaughtered for human consumption…

THE PLAGUE OF ATHENS

As the pigeons coo and the motorbikes roar, we lie on the bed and try to read. I'm trying to read about the history of medicine in ancient Greece. But I'm stuck, like tyres in mud, on the chapter about the terrible plague which ravaged Athens between 430 and 426BC, ending in one stroke the Periclean golden age. It was survived by Thucydides, who left an unsettling account which my book, Helen King's *Greek and Roman Medicine*, paraphrases graphically:

'The disorder started in the head and moved down the body, affecting in turn the eyes, mouth, voice, chest and stomach. If patients survived the retching and vomiting, the disease went on to affect the bowels. Those who did not die could be left with the loss of their fingers and toes, blindness, or loss of memory. The sick felt such extreme fever and thirst, made no better by drinking, that they would jump into tanks of water if they could.'

Thank God we brought those Milton wipes!

48

The Athens plague lasted for over two years and killed a third of the city's population. Thucydides thought it originated in Ethiopia and arrived in Athens via Egypt and Libya, but to this day no one is sure about its provenance or pathology. One theory, though, is that it was an unusually severe type of 'flu exacerbated by bacterial infection...

'Flu.

Avian 'flu.

There is a dead pigeon in our bathroom.

Of the 15 avian influenza virus subtypes currently in existence, the most worrying is H5N1 because of the rapidity of its mutation and its ability to acquire genes from viruses affecting other animal species. Birds that survive the disease continue to excrete the virus for at least ten days, facilitating further transmission.

Influenza pandemics generally occur three to four times each century. The worst in recent history was the 'Spanish' flu pandemic of 1918-19, in which 40 to 50 million people died. But there were also lesser pandemics in 1957-58 and 1968-69. We are due another one.

The Greek physician Hippocrates – of oath fame – is said to have cured the Athenian plague by burning scented wood to ward off the miasma. But did he? He was certainly active in 430BC when the plague began, but beyond that little is known of him. He came from the island of Cos and charged a fee to teach medicine.

He left behind the 60 or so texts known today as 'the Hippocratic corpus', though how many of them he wrote himself remains moot.

Bedside manner is as important to Hippocrates as nitty-gritty stuff like tumour-removal. *On Decorum* advises the doctor to cultivate his patients' trust by dressing modestly and avoiding strong perfumes. *Epidemics* contains the classic diagnostic tip: 'Wax in people's ears; if it is sweet, it foretells death, but if bitter, not.'

It's in the corpus that the first recorded reference to something called hypochondria appears, in an aphorism concerning the treatment of fever: 'If jaundice arise in a fever on the seventh, eleventh or fourteenth day, it is good, unless the right hypochondrium be hard, in which case it is bad.' Here, hypochondrium – hypochondria is the plural – is being used as an anatomical term to refer to a specific area of the lower abdomen: the 'hypo' (under) and 'chondros' (the cartilage of the ribs).

Greek science held that there were four elements – earth, air, fire and water; also that variations in health and temperament were the result of fluctuations in the balance of the body's four controlling 'humours': blood, phlegm, black bile and yellow bile. Black bile – or 'melan chondros' – was supposedly produced by the spleen, located in the left hypochondrium. Hence melancholy people, who suffered from an excess of black bile, were 'splenetic'.

What did this black bile look like? Hildegard of Bingen, writing in the 12th century, had a hunch: 'It is like a slime that is sticky and can be stretched to various lengths.'

The Greeks believed that the lower abdomen – the hypochondria – was the source of all emotional distemper. Galen of Pergamum (129-216AD), Antiquity's other top-dog physician, linked the term to a range of digestive disorders.

Galen knew all about digestion. On one celebrated occasion he removed, then replaced, the intestines of a live ape before a cheering crowd of politicians and intellectuals. Galen also liked to perform public brain surgery on live monkeys, but switched to goats after he started to worry that the expression the monkeys made while he was rooting around in their heads was 'too human'.

Galen thought melancholy was caused by a phenomenon he called 'adust' ('burnt'). Here, a heating of the hypochondriacal organs sent 'some kind of sooty and smoke-like evaporation or some sort of heavy vapours… up from the stomach to the eyes'.

THE ANATOMY OF MELANCHOLY

Gradually, 'hypochondria' becomes synonymous with 'melancholy', though for years the terms resist easy definition as their meanings cross-fertilise. Melancholy can mean sadness, for sure; but it also refers to a range of other conditions including epilepsy.

The bible for melancholics was Robert Burton's 900-page masterpiece *The Anatomy of Melancholy*, first published in 1621. Burton was a reclusive, solitary man who devoted his life to researching and revising the *Anatomy*. Prohibited from marrying by his status as a fellow of Christ Church College, Oxford, he died alone in his college rooms in 1640, having found the single life 'abominable, impious, adulterous and sacrilegious'.

The Anatomy of Melancholy is everything Burton had ever read and thought about decanted gluggingly into a single work ranging across philosophy, astronomy, medicine, politics and literature. Like Laurence Sterne's self-sabotaging comic novel *Tristram Shandy* (1759-67), the *Anatomy* is apparently rambling but actually carefully constructed in neat partitions, each illustrated by a synoptical table. (Sterne drew heavily on the *Anatomy* for *Tristram Shandy*, but the theft passed unnoticed for years, Burton's work having fallen out of print between 1676 and 1800.)

On the book's intricately engraved frontispiece, Burton – or rather Democritus Junior, the pseudonym he uses – identifies several different modes of melancholy, from love-sickness to loneliness and religious obsession. One of these is 'hypochondriacal melancholy'. An explanatory poem, 'The Argument of the Frontispiece', describes a typical sufferer:

> 'Hypochondriacus leans on his arm,
> Wind in his side doth him much harm,
> And troubles him full sore, God knows,
> Much pain he hath and many woes.
> About him pots and glasses lie,
> Newly bought from's Apothecary.
> This Saturn's aspects signify,
> You see them portray'd in the sky.'

So full of examples and symptoms is the *Anatomy* that, for all its charm and brilliance, it is almost impossible to navigate. Some melancholics, we are told, fear that they will go to hell; that every man they meet will rob them; that 'the ground will sinke under them'. Others 'dreame of Hobgoblins'.

And yet hypochondriacal melancholy does have tangible physical symptoms: 'Sharp belchings... fulsome crudities, heat in the bowels, wind and grumbling in the guts... cold sweat...ears ringing, vertigo and giddiness.' There's also an obsession with imaginary illnesses: '[Sufferers] suspect some part or other to be amisse, now their head akes, heart, stomach, spleene, &c. is misaffected, they shall surely have this or that disease.'

Summer 1984. I am at boarding school in Hampshire. It's a Catholic prep school, with a live-in priest and everything. The priest is called Father Douglas. He's very old, with fluffy white hair and giant elephant's ears that go up and down when he chews. He's never looked well, but this term he seems iller than ever – more stooped, with rheumy eyes and a barking cough. We huddle in small groups, whispering the rumour: Father Douglas is about to die.

It's important to watch him closely, in case we miss anything. Never has morning mass been so well attended. We're not forced to go – it's not that hard-line a school; not Jesuit or anything – but go we do, buzzing with unanswerable questions. If a priest dies while saying mass, does that mean he goes to Heaven quicker than if he was, say, eating dinner? Does singing a hymn put a greater strain on the heart than giving a sermon?

Maybe Mr Beadle will know.

Mr Beadle teaches maths, but he used to be a professional footballer. He used to play for Crystal Palace in the late 1950s, and is gloriously easy to divert during lessons; ever eager to relate, once again, how he had all his toenails removed to improve his ball control.

'Did it hurt, sir? When they ripped off your toenails?'

'Of course it did, JJ.' For some reason, Mr Beadle calls me JJ. 'But footballers were tough in those days. Not like this modern lot.'

'Sir?'

'Yes, JJ.'

'Is Father Douglas about to die?'

'What?' Mr Beadle spins round, chalk in fingers. 'Of course not. Wherever did you get that idea?'

So: Mr Beadle doesn't know, or if he does he isn't telling.

Maybe Mr Willis knows.

Mr Willis teaches religious education. Today we are learning about Saint Theresa of Lisieux, a Carmelite nun who was canonised by Pope Pius XI in 1925, a mere 28 years after her death at 24. She became famous for her extreme piety and self-denial, proof of which may be found in her 'spiritual autobiography', *Story of a Soul.*

Mr Willis is completely in love with Saint Theresa of Lisieux. He goes on and on about her. He even hands out little cards with her photo on. Our first impression is that she is quite shockingly ugly; but maybe this is unfair. No one looks great in a wimple.

The lesson drags on. Mr Willis explains that life in a Carmelite nunnery was austere and demanding. But though Sister Theresa was physically frail, she threw herself into working in the kitchen, and even acted the part of Joan of

Arc in a play the nuns staged.

In 1895, Sister Theresa wrote that she had heard, 'as it was, a far-off murmur announcing the coming of the Bridegroom'.

'Now,' says Mr Willis. 'What do you think she meant by this?'

There is a collective shrugging of shoulders.

Eventually, someone asks: 'Did she get a letter from an old boyfriend?'

'No,' says Mr Willis.

Another hand goes up. 'Did she get special permission to leave the convent to go to a wedding?'

'No,' says Mr Willis. He looks at his watch. 'Come on. You can do better than this.'

Oh no we can't.

He sighs explosively. 'Well if you're all going

> **The tuberculosis virus can live for months in the dark in dried saliva.**

to be so *useless*... She'd started bleeding from her mouth. Haemorrhaging, it's called. Saint Theresa was in the early stages of tuberculosis. She knew it would kill her in the end, so when she talked about the Bridegroom she meant Jesus Christ, who she knew she would meet in Heaven.'

He goes on: 'Saint Theresa saw illness as something to celebrate – as something unique she had been given by

God: a spiritual trial. Though of course, she knew well that no hardship she suffered could possibly match what Jesus had suffered on the cross.'

This is yucky on *so many levels*, it's hard to keep track.

Time for a change of subject.

'Sir, is Father Douglas about to die?'

***

Mr Willis asks me to stay behind after the class. He tells me off for asking an inappropriate question and bans me from watching *Top of the Pops* that evening, but I don't care because it's only David Bowie at number one again and I haven't yet learned to love David Bowie.

In any case, there are important developments. Pearson, who is younger than us but has a cool Walkman with Dolby noise reduction and two headphone sockets, rushes into our dormitory. We're the first people he's told: Father Douglas has a bandaged hand. The official line is that he has bad arthritis in his wrist, but we know better.

'He's got stigmata,' says Pearson. 'Like Padre Pio.'

Stigmata are marks on your body like Christ's wounds. You usually get them in the places where He was nailed to the cross – the hands, the feet; or around the head where the Crown of Thorns would have sat. You wouldn't get them on your shin, though you might in your side because that's where the Roman soldier stuck his spear.

We know about Padre Pio from *Mysteries of the Un-explained*, a book which Bartlett's father gave him. There are photos of him – Padre Pio, not Bartlett's father – where you can see his scabby hands outstretched and the congregation leaning forward going 'oooh'.

Padre Pio was an Italian priest who died in 1968. He was – is – the world's most famous stigmatic. On September 20, 1918, he was kneeling before a large crucifix when the marks appeared on him for the first time. A vision appeared beside him of a man whose hands, feet and side were dripping blood. When the man disappeared, Padre Pio looked at his own hands and saw that blood was pouring from them. At this point he fell into a kind of trance. 'All the internal and external senses and even the very faculties of my soul were immersed in indescribable stillness,' he wrote to his spiritual advisor, Padre Benedetto.

At the Vatican's insistence, Padre Pio took to conducting mass wearing mittens to hide his bleeding hands. Those who smelt his wounds reported a scent of perfume, the 'odour of sanctity'.

But back to Father Douglas. Someone asks the crucial question: 'Were the bandages stained with blood?'

Pearson frowns. 'I don't know. I didn't notice.'

There is tutting and shaking of heads.

We resolve to look more carefully tomorrow.

DISEASE OF THE LEARNED

Thanks to Robert Burton, hypochondria soon became a signifier of 'artistic temperament'. To be melancholy was to belong to an elite club, though a poor person suffering similar symptoms would have been regarded as sullen and awkward.

A common cause of hypochondriacal melancholy was deception in love. A collection of songs by one Timothy Tulip ('of Fidlers-Hall in Cuckoldshire'), published in 1732, bears the title *The Merry Mountebank; or, the Humourous Quack-Doctor: Being a certain, safe and speedy CURE, for that Heart-Breaking DISTEMPER, commonly call'd or known by the Name of Hypochondriac-Melancholy*. The songs are subtly bawdy hymns to wine and women. 'A Two-Part Song on a Bowl of Punch' goes:

'The Jolly Bowl does glad my Soul
The flowing Liquor cheers my Heart…'

A few pages on, the outcome of 'As Celia near a Fountain lay…' – in which snoozing Celia snares the attention of a randy shepherd called Damon – might be predicted:

'Damon embrac'd the lucky Hit
And flew into her Arms
He took her in the yielding Fit
And rifl'd all her Charms.'

'Hypochondriack Passion should be called the Disease of the Learned,' wrote B Mandeville in *A Treatise of the Hypochondriack and Hysterick Diseases* (1730), adding that it was commonest in those who, 'either by Estate, Benefices, or Employments have a sufficient Revenue to make themselves easie'.

The other suspect category was writers, obliged to submit themselves daily to the unpredictable force of their imaginations. In Samuel Johnson's philosophical novel *Rasselas* (1759), the sage Imlac warns that this is a recipe for worry and depression:

'To indulge the power of fiction, and send imagination out upon the wing, is often the sport of those who delight too much in silent speculation... He who has nothing external that can divert him must find pleasure in his own thoughts, and must conceive himself what he is not; for who is pleased with what he is?'

Certainly not Johnson's biographer, James Boswell.

Between 1777 and 1783, Boswell wrote a series of essays for the *London Magazine* under the byline 'The Hypochondriack'. A nervy, depressive character ('I snatch gratifications,' he wrote, 'but have no comfort'), Boswell was unable to take routine ailments in his stride. Having caught 'Signor Gonorrhoea' from one of the many prostitutes who indulged his penchant for alfresco sex, he was tormented by nightmares: 'I lay in direful apprehension that my testicle, which formerly was ill, was again swelled. I dreamed that Douglas [his physician] stood by me and said, "This is a damned difficult case."'

Dr Johnson, himself a hypochondriac, advised his young friend to keep occupied, take more exercise and drink less at night. But you sense that Boswell was too addicted to the idea of hypochondria as a badge of artistic sensitivity to pay much attention. In an essay from 1778, he invokes Aristotle's belief that melancholy is 'the concomitant of distinguished genius', adding: 'We Hypochondriacks may be glad to accept of this compliment from so great a master of human nature, and to console ourselves in the hour of gloomy distress, by thinking that our sufferings mark our superiority.'

NATURE'S WATER

On Sundays at school we do Scouts. We get to cook in the woods behind the school – to fry sausages in pans heated by real flames from a real fire. We wrap potatoes in tin foil and place them in the embers, because if you do this and leave them long enough then they bake. (In fact, they never cook properly because we never leave them long enough because we don't know how long 'long enough' is.)

This Sunday is better than last Sunday because it is hotter, plus Brigstock has brought his water purifier so we can drink water from streams and rivers and ponds like we would if we were in the army.

The water purifier is like a big canvas sock. Brigstock ordered it from an army supplies catalogue. He wants to join the army when he's old enough. He says everyone should join the army – that if you don't you're not doing your duty. Unfashionably precise in speech and dress, Brigstock is a bit of a laughing stock. At the same time, we always defer to him on matters military and tactical because his father is a sergeant major.

Sometimes Major Brigstock comes to school events wearing his uniform. He has a moustache and a booming posh voice. Once I was helping at Prize Giving and I had to serve him sandwiches from a silver platter and when he took one he went 'Ra-ther!' and I went back and told everyone and the next day when Brigstock came into the classroom we saluted him and kept going 'Ra-ther! Ra-ther!' but he cried so we stopped.

Brigstock takes his water purifier and goes off to find some water to purify. He says it's important to drink lots of water when you eat sausages because sausages are very salty and if you were in a combat zone in say a desert and you ate too much salty food you would get

The American Institute for Cancer Research (AICR) warns that barbecues are a huge health risk. Not just because of the risk of food poisoning from undercooked meat: the grilling of 'muscle meats' such as steak typically causes fat to drip on to the hot coals or stones. This burnt fat forms carcinogens called heterocyclic amines (HCAs), which are reabsorbed by the food when the smoke and flames char the meat.

dehydrated more quickly and so be more likely to die.

While Brigstock is gone, Stoddart and I fry the sausages. They keep sticking to the pan, so we keep adding more lard. The fat sizzles and spits and smokes. After five minutes, Stoddart says: 'I think they're done.'

'What? Really?'

'Yeah. The skin's all black.'

'But they're pink inside.'

'Doesn't matter. What matters is to eat quickly. Brigstock says that in a combat zone, speed is of the essence or the enemy might eat your rations.'

We agree that this would be a bad thing.

Brigstock returns just as we're tucking in. He looks elated. He's filled the purifier with water from a puddle. 'I sort of scooped it up,' he explains. He hangs it on a branch and we watch as surprisingly clear-looking water drip-drip-drips into the mug underneath.

'That's nature's water,' says Brigstock, proudly. 'The most pure water you'll ever drink.'

There isn't much of it, but we get about three mud-tasting mouthfuls each.

THE ENGLISH MALADY

The Scottish philosopher David Hume was diagnosed with Disease of the Learned at the age of 19. One can only imagine the expression on the face of the doctor to whom Hume presented his main symptom: an excessively watery mouth. Perhaps the prescription is revealing? Hume told George Cheyne, author of *The English Malady* (1733), that he 'went under a Course of Bitters, & Anti-hysteric Pills, drunk an English Pint of Claret Wine every Day, and rode eight or ten Scotch Miles. This I continu'd for about seven Months after.' By which time, you might think, he would have been too exhausted and hungover to notice how he was feeling.

Cheyne himself was a curious fellow – a London-dwelling Scot prone to alternating bouts of binge-eating and crash-dieting. At his largest he weighed 300 pounds and came close to crushing the horse he sat on; but a meatless diet quickly slimmed him down again. The only satisfactory cure Cheyne found for his persistent headaches and giddiness was wintering in Bath, where he could relax and take the water, far from the capital's gastronomic temptations. Cheyne believed that a combination of spicy foods and intemperate living was the culprit: 'Since our [ie, England's] wealth has increased and our Navigation has been extended, we have ransacked all the Parts of the Globe to bring together its whole Stock of Materials for Riot, Luxury and to provoke Excess.'

(Boswell devoted several of his 'Hypochondriack' columns to food – specifically the difference between French and English cuisine – but his thoughts never strayed far from sex: 'There is something I think particularly indelicate and disgusting in the idea of a cook-maid,' he wrote, randomly. 'Imagination can easily cherish a fondness for a pretty chambermaid or dairymaid, but one is revolted by the greasiness and scorching connected with the wench who toils in the kitchen.')

Food is also an issue for Robert Whytt in (deep breath) *Observations on the Nature, Cause and Cure of Those Disorders Which are Commonly Called Nervous, Hypochondriacal or Hysterical* (1764). Certain illnesses, he thought, were the result of a 'sympathy of the nerves' whereby a sensation in one part of the body triggered a symptom elsewhere. 'The smell of grateful food makes the saliva flow when one is hungry,' he declared, incontestably, observing that this caused an 'irritation of the windpipe' which might lead to 'coughing, or convulsive motion of the muscles employed in expiration'.

Whytt felt that some people were simply more sensitive to physical maladies than others. Artistic types, obviously, fell into this category; so too all women and children. But this sensitivity could be acquired, or even a scar-like legacy of illness or other trauma. 'Long and repeated fevers, profuse haemorrhages, great fatigue, excessive and long continued grief, luxurious living, and want of exercise, may increase and even bring on such a delicate state of the nervous system,' he wrote.

The last hurrah for the idea that feeling inexplicably rough might have a physical basis came in 1807, with former Royal Navy physician Thomas Trotter's *A View of the Nervous Temperament*. Like Cheyne, and indeed Galen, Trotter's focus was the digestive system ('anatomists have discovered an unusual share of nerves about the upper orifice of the stomach...'), and at certain points he seems to anticipate

Campylobacters are the spiral-shaped bacteria that most commonly cause diarrhoea in humans. Although a fatal outcome from campylo-bacteriosis is rare, post-infection complications can include the neurological disorder Guillain-Barré syndrome, a polio-like form of paralysis.

contemporary thinking about Irritable Bowel Syndrome. At others, though, he comes on like the crusty old reactionary he was, railing against the moral laxity of city life:

'Amidst the great effeminacy of manners, that is rapidly consuming the very spiritual and physical strength of this age, what may ultimately annihilate all that is great in the character of the Britons, it is somewhat consoling to observe that the seamen of the navy, that bulwark of our liberties, will be the last of the community to feel the effect of those enervating customs.'

In other words, hypochondria is for girls.

SORT OF A FUNNY PAIN

It is the middle of the night. People keep getting out of bed. Running to the bathroom. Being sick. Then huffing and sighing and trying not to cry because crying is wet.

Who are these people? Why, they are Brigstock and Stoddart and me. Brigstock signals and we follow him out of the dormitory and into the hall.

'I've been sick about four million times,' I say, untruthfully. 'That water...'

'It wasn't the water,' snaps Brigstock. 'The water was pure.

It was your fucking sausages.'

We have recently discovered that swearing makes you sound really hard.

Stoddart says, 'Maybe we should wake matron?'

There is a silence. I know that all three of us are, in our heads, filling this silence in the same way. We are filling it with images of Mr Beadle wincing as he squishes his bruised, deformed feet into his football boots. Of Saint Theresa as she holds a handkerchief to her mouth to catch the coughed-up specks of blood. Of Padre Pio and his weeping palms (though not that devious old charlatan Father Douglas, who we've decided is only wearing bandages to make us *think* he's stigmatic).

They didn't complain. They withstood the torment. It made them better people. Better Catholics. And we all want to be better Catholics, don't we?

Stoddart is the first to speak. 'I think we should wake matron,' he says.

'Me too,' I say.

'Honestly,' sighs Brigstock. 'You are so fucking wet. You wouldn't last two minutes in the SAS.'

SOME SLIGHT AILMENT

By 1849, the year someone calling himself MRCS published

Confessions of a Hypochondriac: or The Adventures of a Hyp In Search of Health, the hypochondriac had become a bit of a joke. MRCS is constantly consulting different doctors and receiving different, contradictory diagnoses ('It seemed as if these accomplished gentlemen were ruled to overrule each other'). He tries homeopathy for his 'psoric malady', taking 'less than the millionth part of a grain of the pansy violet (viola tricolor), which was subsequently superseded by the billionth of a grain of sulphur'.

It was the Victorians' misfortune to live on the cusp of a new age of medicine – an age in which germ theory and penicillin would transform the way diseases were thought about and treated. All around them, important advances were being made, like the discovery of vaccines for smallpox and rabies, and the invention of the stethoscope. As the Empire expanded, so did people's sense of what was possible medically. They expected much from the doctors they paid through the nose to see, but most of these practitioners were charlatans.

Over-the-counter remedies, too, were skilfully advertised but worthless even as placebos. Beechams Pills, for 'nervous or bilious disorders, sick headache, giddiness, fullness and swelling after meals' and everything else besides, contained only aloes, a purgative soap. The opening of London's first underground railway, the Metropolitan line, prompted much bellyaching about the impact on passengers' health of the steam trains' emissions, or 'choke damp'. Opportunistic chemists did a roaring trade in something calling itself Designated Metropolitan Mixture, probably laudanum.

The creation of a proper sewage system for London in the 1870s did much to preserve the city from water-borne epidemics, but by this time the century had seen several waves of infectious diseases – two flu epidemics between 1831 and 1833, as well as the first outbreak of cholera, which killed 52,000. There was another attack of cholera between 1836 and 1842; also epidemics of typhoid and typhus.

Little surprise that Londoners were jittery about their health. When we first meet Jerome, George and William Samuel Harris in Jerome K Jerome's *Three Men in a Boat* (1889), they are sitting around, 'talking about how bad we were – from a medical point of view I mean, of course'. Jerome, especially, convinces himself that he has any disease he reads about:

'I remember going to the British Museum one day to read up the treatment for some slight ailment of which I had a touch – hay fever, I fancy it was. I got down the book, and read all I came to read; and then, in an unthinking moment, I idly turned the leaves, and began to indolently study diseases, generally. I forget which was the first distemper I plunged into – some fearful, devastating scourge, I know – and, before

I had glanced down half the list of "premonitory symptoms",
it was borne in upon me that I had fairly got it.'

Jerome decides that he is suffering from every disease listed in the encyclopedia – apart from housemaid's knee. He goes to see his doctor, who hits him over the chest ('a cowardly thing to do, I call it'), butts him on the side of the head, then writes him the following prescription:

'1lb beefsteak, with
1pt bitter beer every six hours.
1 ten-mile walk every morning.
1 bed at 11 sharp every night.
And don't stuff up your head with things you don't understand.'

KIND OF TREMULOUS

Traditionally, hypochondria was a male condition. Female hypochondriacs were judged to be suffering from 'hysteria', from the Greek for womb 'hystera'. The ancient Greeks believed that the womb floated around the body causing trouble wherever it stopped.

A common manifestation of hysteria was 'neurasthenia' – a state of nervous distress for which no organic cause could be found. The Victorians fetishised disease as enthusiastically as they feared it, and our sense of neurasthenia as a female-specific disorder owes much to the fragile, usually consumptive heroines of novels like Henri Murger's *Scenes de la Vie de Boheme* (1851), the basis for Puccini's opera *La Boheme*.

Yet the man who first identified neurasthenia, the American physician and neurologist George Miller Beard, had no sense of it as gender-specific. He called it 'American nervousness', and blamed it on the pressures of life in an industrialised society. Men, who increasingly faced a long commute to work where they would have to wrestle with new-fangled technologies like the telephone, were as likely to suffer from it as women.

That neurasthenia was a rather vague catch-all term is obvious from Beard's list of its defining symptoms, compiled in 1869: headaches; deafness; scalp tenderness; morbid fears and other phobias; mild depression; sleeplessness; blushing; excessive sweating; cramps; heart palpitations; increased ticklishness; cold extremities; tooth decay; excessive yawning; vaginismus; impotence; and, wonderfully, 'tremulousness'.

You okay? You seem a bit off-colour.

Yeah. I've been feeling kind of tremulous all day. It'll pass...

Like its companion disorder hypochondria, neurasthenia was common among intellectuals and other professional sensitives; but the degree of tolerance extended varied wildly according to the progressiveness of your social circle. On the one hand, the trade in tranquillising potions (usually laudanum) kept many a rogue doctor afloat. Wealthy valetudinarians were routinely bundled off to health spas to be pampered and massaged. They might go to Bath to take the waters, though not everyone was convinced of their efficacy. 'The water contains nothing but a little salt, and calcarious earth, mixed in such inconsiderable proportion, as can have very little, if any, effect on the animal oeconomy,' wrote novelist and doctor Tobias Smollett in *Humphry Clinker*. 'This being the case, I think the man deserves to be fitted with a cap and bells, who, for such a paltry advantage as this spring affords, sacrifices his precious time, which might be employed in taking more effectual remedies.'

MRCS visits Malvern and Cheltenham in search of a 'water cure', but fails to find satisfaction. 'After a day or two I ceased to mend, and tired my physician again and again with the strange tale of my perverse, unintelligible, and inexplicable illness, and at last, to get rid of me I suppose, he advised me to travel. This is the usual way of disposing of a patient of my class.'

Inspired by a friend's recommendation, MRCS visits a bath in Brighton and treats himself to a massage ('that eastern luxury'). A 'huge Egyptian' shampoos him and cracks his joints 'like a whip': 'When I found him sitting on my chest, as if on a squab, I merely smiled in his face, when in ordinary, I believe,

73

I should have smitten him seriously on the cheek.'

Over in New York, Beard experimented with an early form of electro-convulsive therapy. But one person's neurasthenia was another's malingering, and some cures were positively brutal, especially if you were young and female. For many doctors, as Elaine Showalter explains, 'the goal was to isolate the patient from her family support systems, unmask her deceitful stratagems, coerce her into surrendering her symptoms, and finally overcome her self-centredness'.

Doctors such as these practised 'observant neglect': what Showalter characterises as deliberate indifference to a patient's expectations of sympathy; also physical violence like slapping and suppression of the supraorbital nerve just above the eye. At Cheltenham Ladies College in 1889, the standard cure for hysterical fits was to dose patients with laxatives, then throw freezing cold water over them.

The justification for this harshness was a growing suspicion among doctors that hypochondria and neurasthenia were symptoms of moral weakness. But the Victorians' fear of disease was heightened by the knowledge that, were they to contract cholera or typhoid, nothing any doctor could do would prevent death. In some cases this seems to have licensed a resigned acceptance of illness which can look self-indulgent.

Mr Fairlie in Wilkie Collins's *The Woman in White* (1859-

60) is a classic patient-as-tyrant. Hero Walter Hartright dislikes him on sight, considering his 'frail, languidly-fretful, over-refined look' to be 'unpleasantly delicate in its association with a man' and his hypochondria to be a 'selfish affectation'. Anything and everything – light, a visitor moving across the room, the slightest sound – is 'exquisitely painful' to Mr Fairlie: '"Gently with the curtains, please – the slightest noise from them goes through me like a knife."'

The behaviour of an entire household could be dictated by the hypochondriac at its centre. 'In my grandparents' house it was a distinction and a mournful pleasure to be ill,' wrote Charles Darwin's grand-daughter, Gwen Raverat. 'This was partly because my grandfather was always ill, and his children adored him and were inclined to imitate him; and partly because it was so delightful to be pitied and nursed by my grandmother...

> **New diseases that emerged or were identified between 1980 and 1993:**
>
> **1980: Toxic Shock Syndrome**
> **1981: AIDS**
> **1982: Eschericia Coli 0157:H7**
> **1984: Brazilian purpuric fever**
> **1986: Human ehrlichiosis**
> **1989: Venezuelan haemorrhagic fever**
> **1989: Toxic shock-like syndrome**
> **1993: Hantavirus pulmonary syndrome**
>
> Source: *Plague's Progress*, Arno Karlen (Indigo 1995)

At Down [House], illness was considered normal.'

THE MAN WHO COLLECTED BEETLES

Charles Darwin was born in Shrewsbury on February 12, 1809, the second youngest of six children. He was a poor student who later admitted: 'School as a means of education to me was simply a blank.' Sent to Edinburgh by his doctor father to study medicine, he made little progress and junked the course halfway through. Fearing Charles would live out his days an 'idle sporting man', his father suggested he become a clergyman.

Darwin agreed. He went up to Cambridge, as trainee clergymen did, but spent most of his time shooting and hunting and drinking and playing cards in the company of 'dissipated low-minded young men'. Yet he had a saving passion: collecting beetles.

Through this hobby he met Professor of Botany John Stevens Henslow, the man who would transform Darwin's life and more besides by informing him that one Captain FitzRoy, who was about to embark on an important scientific expedition, had agreed to find space in his cabin for a young naturalist who was happy not to be paid.

Captain FitzRoy's ship was called the Beagle. It was quite a big ship – a ten-gun brig weighing 242 tons. Darwin boarded it on October 25, 1831. From the start he was miserable with seasickness, but otherwise notably active – an enthusiastic collector of animals, fossils, rocks and plants which he shipped straight back to Henslow in Cambridge. (He lacked the talent to draw them himself.) When the ship docked – the expedition's aim was to explore the coasts of Patagonia, Tierra del Fuego, Chile, Peru and the Pacific Islands – Darwin was among the first to saddle up and set off to explore the interior. He quickly acquired a reputation as one of the hardiest men on board, not to mention an able mountaineer.

Its five-year voyage over, the Beagle anchored at Falmouth on October 2, 1836. Darwin later wrote that it was in July 1837 that he 'opened [his] first note-book for facts in relation to the Origin of Species, about which [he] had long reflected, and never ceased working for the next twenty years'. This coincides almost exactly with his first complaints of heart palpitations.

In October 1837 he turned down the Secretaryship of the Geological Society because of the stress it would involve. On January 29, 1839 he married his cousin, Emma, daughter of Josiah Wedgwood. The marriage was famously long and happy, but also the trigger for massive changes in Darwin's lifestyle and outlook. At the age of 32, it seems the former explorer consciously recast himself as an invalid who was able to function only in total social isolation. He moved with Emma to Down House in a remote corner of the Kent countryside, where he cultivated an almost comically neurasthenic persona.

Emma's whole day revolved around Charles; she was on constant call lest he wish to be read to or accompanied on a walk. His son, Sir Francis Darwin, remembers: 'After dinner he never stayed in the room, and used to apologise by saying he was an old woman who must be allowed to leave with the ladies… Half an hour more or less of conversation would make to him the difference of a sleepless night and of the loss perhaps of half the next day's work.'

Charles himself corroborated this assessment in a letter to a Mr Fox on March 28, 1843: 'I cannot dine out or receive visitors except relations with whom I can pass some time after dinner in silence.'

Travelling into London exhausted him. 'I find most unfortunately for myself,' he wrote to FitzRoy on March 31, 1843, 'that the little excitement of breaking out of my quiet routine so generally knocks me up that I am able to do scarcely anything when in London.'

Initially, Darwin's heart caused him the most concern. But before long his nervous system became affected so that his hands trembled, and his stomach played up. He wrote to Sir William Jackson Hooker: 'I believe I have not had one whole day or rather night without my stomach having been grossly disordered during the last three years and most days great prostration of strength; thank you for your kindness; many of my friends, I believe, think me a hypochondriac.'

In this, Darwin was correct. The finest doctors of the day found nothing organically wrong with him, and his neighbour, the anatomy specialist Sir Arthur Keith, came close to diagnosing hypochondria when he wrote that 'the voluntary part of [Darwin's] brain seemed to have too easy and too free an access to his involuntary part'. On those rare occasions when he turned to his father for advice and support, he was invariably disappointed: 'I told him of my dreadful numbness in my finger ends, and all the sympathy I could get was "Yes-yes-exactly-tut-tut, neuralgic, exactly, yes, yes!",' he told Emma in a letter in October 1843.

A variety of explanations for Darwin's condition have been proposed over the years: that he was suffering from gout, or brucellosis, or paroxysmal tachycardia... The most outré theory is Chagas's disease, which some believe Darwin contracted after being bitten on the *Beagle* by 'the Benchuca, a species of Reduvius, the great black bug of the Pampas', though this has been discredited. Had Darwin suffered from Chagas's disease, there would be more substantial evidence of progressive heart failure. As it was, he would frequently walk several miles a day unhindered by pain or breathlessness, swinging a heavy stick as he went. A coronary did eventually kill him in 1882, but by then he was 73 – ancient by Victorian standards – so this falls within the compass of 'natural causes'.

What was wrong with Darwin? Today, assuming a battery of tests showed up nothing, he might well be diagnosed with 'conversion disorder', one of the oldest psychological illnesses on the menu – the kind of thing the neurologist Jean-Martin Charcot was teaching his star pupil Sigmund Freud to cure using hypnosis in early-twentieth-century Paris. It's where physical symptoms occur in the absence of organic pathology – because they are an expression of an underlying emotional conflict. A typical example would be someone who was afraid of singing in public losing her voice. One health website estimates that 34 per cent of Americans experience a conversion disorder in the course of their lifetimes – though 90 per cent recover within a month.

Conversion disorder is a sub-species of 'somatoform disorder'. When doctors decide that a person's hypochondria has moved beyond the stage of being amusing, then annoying, then infuriating – has, in other words, shuffled on to the same axis as obsessive-compulsive disorder, body dysmorphic disorder and major depression – they start talking about somatoform disorder: a morbidly excessive awareness of ordinary bodily processes. The sufferer lies in bed, listening to his stomach digesting food. He times his bowel movements and the intervals between them.

When things get this bad, the prescription is either one of

the SSRI class of antidepressants such as Prozac or cognitive behavioural therapy. This is all about teaching patients to rationalise the threat of disease in their lives, and to stop associating symptoms with sickness – to realise that it's not possible to feel well all the time. (We touched on this earlier.) While undergoing treatment, patients are forbidden from examining their bodies for signs of disease, or from 'researching' illnesses in books or on the internet.

Darwin clearly felt that his preoccupation with illness impaired his life, even if, unconsciously, he enjoyed being ill. But where would he fall on the spectrum? And if we assume that he did indeed suffer from conversion disorder, what sub-conscious conflict was he trying to convert, and why?

The religious implications of evolutionary theory worried away at Darwin while he worked on it. To Hooker he remarked that *The Origin of Species* was 'a very presumptuous work, and I know no one individual who would not say a very foolish one'. He had never intended to be at the vanguard of an attack on Christianity, even if his own faith had lapsed on the Beagle, where he came to feel that 'the Old Testament was no more to be trusted than the sacred books of the Hindoos'.

Darwin hated conflict and controversy. Yet he knew that *The Origin of Species* would be savaged by the church and make him an intellectual outcast. The year after it was finally published in 1859, it was denounced by the Bishop of Oxford, 'Soapy' Sam Wilberforce, at a particularly tumultuous meeting of the British Association which moved Darwin to observe: 'I am glad I was not at Oxford, for I should have been overwhelmed, with my stomach in its present state... I would as soon have died as tried to answer the Bishop in such an assembly.'

As Ralph Colp reveals in his account of Darwin's illnesses, 'To Be An Invalid', he had worrying precedents in mind: 'Darwin had read how the French naturalist Buffon

> **The bacteria that causes 'strep throat' – group A streptococcus – is also responsible for necrotising fasciitis, aka the 'flesh-eating bug'.**

had been forced to recant his theory about the history of the earth because it had been judged to contradict Scripture; he had witnessed how a member of the Edinburgh Plinian Society had expressed materialist ideas about the nature of organisms and the mind, and then had these ideas suppressed by the Society.'

Were Darwin's illnesses a physical manifestation of this worry? If so, it's odd that he found he was able to work on his theory even when he was too ill to work on anything else. Perhaps his illnesses were entirely invented – an attempt to regulate his family and social life so that it remained subordinate to his professional life? Darwin, who knew a paradox when he saw one, certainly recognised the benefits of having a weak constitution, admitting later on in his life: 'I know well that my head would have failed years ago had not my stomach saved me from a minute's over-work.'

DARWIN VS MR WOODHOUSE

How much free time did Darwin have on the *Beagle?* Did he have time to read novels when he wasn't collecting fossils and throwing up? If so, did he ever read Jane Austen's *Emma,* published in 1816?

I only ask because the hypochondriacal persona Darwin affected throughout his life recalls one of Austen's best loved characters – Emma's crotchety father, Mr Woodhouse.

Like Darwin, Mr Woodhouse has a 'horror of late hours and large dinner parties' which made him 'unfit for any acquaintance, but such as would visit him on his own terms'. He is fussy about food, approving the ingestion of little beyond a very softly boiled egg ('not unwholesome') and a bowl of thin gruel. The cake at Miss Taylor's wedding makes him bilious: 'His own stomach could bear nothing rich, and he would never believe other people to be different from himself.'

Out of this egotism, however, flutters a kind of empathy. Indeed, where Mr Woodhouse differs from Darwin is in his concern for other people's health as well as his own: he is constantly fussing over Emma – even though she 'hardly knew what indisposition was' – and expresses 'very genuine unmixed anxiety' as to how foppish Frank Churchill, whom he dislikes, could have spent two nights on the road without catching cold.

Significantly, the word Austen uses to describe Mr Woodhouse is not 'hypochondriac' – which, as we know, was current at the time and so available to her – but 'valetudinarian'. The difference, slight but crucial, is one to which Austen obsessives are minutely attuned. A valetudinarian, according to the Oxford English Dictionary, is 'a person in weak health, esp. one who is constantly concerned with his own ailments; an invalid'. In other words, Mr Woodhouse is *actually ill* and not being satirised, unlike the tedious Mrs Churchill, one of whose nervous seizures delays her nephew Frank's arrival at Box Hill.

So what is wrong with him? Ted Bader, an Austen enthusiast who also happens to be Associate Clinical Professor at the University of Colorado Health Sciences Center, thinks Mr Woodhouse might have hypothyroidism, a hormonal disorder of the thyroid gland which can lead to feelings of 'coldness, mental nervousness and skeletal weakness'.

Bader is also a CS Lewis fan, and points out that the Cambridge don and author of the Narnia books, who claimed to have read Austen's novel 12 times, considered Mr Woodhouse to be 'the most sensible character in *Emma*'. I can only agree.

On the subject of hypothyroidism, though, I'm less convinced. One of the condition's most noticeable symptoms is a goitre – a huge and protuberant swelling in the neck where the thyroid gland has become enlarged. A writer of Austen's descriptive subtlety would surely have alluded to the thing somewhere in the course of a 400-page novel, no matter how inappropriate the context.

Cupping his goitre with his left hand, Mr Woodhouse rose from his chair.

'Do take care not to catch cold,' said Mr Woodhouse, whose goitre looked especially disgusting today – all veiny and glistening.

TOP THREE WORRIES FOR TODAY

1. Pins and needles

I keep getting it in my leg when I'm sitting at my desk. Maybe I'm just sitting awkwardly? Compressing a nerve? Or maybe it's Guillain-Barré syndrome, a rare nerve disorder which starts with pins and needles and progresses rapidly to muscle weakness and then paralysis and then needing a respirator to breathe and then death, probably...

2. Forgetting what things are called

In the verbal tests that showed the novelist Iris Murdoch was suffering from Alzheimer's, she was unable to name a kangaroo when it was pictured, describing it instead as a 'beautiful creature that jumps'. Today at work I asked Dave who sits opposite me, 'Can you pass the thing? The clicky black paper thing?' He passed me the stapler without comment.

3. Hiccups

I never normally get hiccups, but I did yesterday. I got a full-blown attack lasting in excess of seven minutes. (Time it: it's longer than you think.) I did the drinking-water-backwards thing but the water went down the wrong way and I choked and some person I'd never met before decided to play the have-a-go hero and started thumping me on the back which made me lurch forward and hit my head on a shelf. Hiccups are the ripples that warn of an impending health tsunami. They can signify an oncoming aortic aneurysm; kidney failure, too; but mostly cancer of the lung, diaphragm, pancreas, liver and/or stomach.

IMAGINARY DISEASES VS DISEASES OF THE IMAGINATION

World War One had a huge impact on attitudes towards

nervous disorders, bequeathing us the concept of 'shell-shock' – a term invented in 1914 by a Cambridge laboratory psychologist, Dr Charles S Myers, so that damaged soldiers returning from the Western Front would not suffer the unmanly indignity of being branded 'hysterical' or 'neurasthenic'. But the Great War's effects ranged far beyond the army, out across the general populace. 'The nerve-strain to which the majority of workers in all belligerent countries have been subjected is already beginning to assert its sinister influence,' declared Ivo Geikie Cobb in *A Manual of Neurasthenia* (1920).

Cobb's attempts to differentiate between 'hypochondria', 'neurasthenia' and 'hysteria' only emphasise the arbitrariness of the distinctions. He followed the prevailing wisdom in regarding hysterics as primarily female and hypochondriacs male. Meanwhile, he wrote, 'hypochondriacal ideas are seen in many cases of neurasthenia; and it not infrequently happens that they tend to mask the real nature of the malady'. Hypochondria he declared 'very rare under 30', and most common in those who lived a 'solitary, sedentary life'. He concluded: 'It is not usual for suicide to end the career.'

Gradually, ideas from the newfangled discipline of psychiatry percolated their way into general medical practice. The notion that the subconscious might be to blame for phobias and other functional derangements was embraced by LS Barnes, the Hertfordshire GP of whom Doris Armitage's *A Challenge to Neurasthenia* (1929) is partly a hagiography.

There was a big difference, Barnes held, between an imaginary disease and a disease of the imagination. He was particularly effective at treating hypochondria. 'One patient, disturbed by the discovery of a small lump, became convinced that this was cancer,' Armitage remembers, 'and the assurances of two doctors that it was harmless failed to carry any lasting conviction.' Barnes's tactic was to encourage the woman to visualise her subconscious as distinct from her – as a deceitful, unscrupulous alter ego. 'He [ie, her subconscious] can hand you bits of things that without context or real knowledge will appear to confirm your fears. But they do not make fact. Why believe this sort of person?'

Barnes's faith in the efficacy of a talking cure for hypochondria is momentous. It suggests that sufferers are at the mercy of processes beyond their control, and that they should be pitied and helped, not punished. His approach was supremely rational and logical. Often patients would say to him something like, 'Yes doctor, very interesting. I can see how what you're saying would help someone else. But my case, and my symptoms, are real, so it doesn't apply to me.' At this, 'he would lean back in his chair and laugh at you. "Of course you believe it is real," he would say; "if you didn't, would it have any hold over you?"

The word 'neurasthenia' may have fallen into disuse, but the kind of conditions which would once have been classed as neurasthenic are still very much with us.

Chronic fatigue syndrome (CFS) or myalgic encephalomyelitis (ME) is a debilitating, flu-like condition whose first recorded appearance was at Los Angeles County General Hospital in 1934. Patients reported muscle pain, lethargy, memory lapses, difficulty concentrating and an inability to walk even short distances without feeling exhausted. Approximately 200 members of the hospital's staff contracted the disease; over half of them were still unable to return to work six months later.

> **Viruses play a role in 15 to 20 per cent of human cancers.**

January 2002 was an important month for the estimated 240,000 people in the UK who sufferer from CFS/ME. A working party set up by Sir Liam Donaldson, the chief medical officer, concluded that CFS/ME was not an imaginary illness, but a chronic and treatable condition. Use of the derogatory expression 'yuppie flu' to describe it was banned. CFS/ME sufferers had for too long been 'dismissed as hypochondriacs and urged to get better on their own', said Donaldson. It was now time for doctors to accept that they were not malingerers and treat them as such.

As a feature by Jerome Burn in the *Guardian* (March 30, 2002) revealed, all was not as clear-cut as it seemed: six members of the working group had resigned in protest just before publication. And rather than be happy that their malady had been officially recognised, CFS/ME activists were furious at the way Donaldson's report fudged the issue of whether CFS/ME had a physical rather than a psychological basis.

There are two camps: those who think CFS/ME is a form of psychoneurosis; and those like Malcolm Hooper, a professor emeritus from Sunderland University, who believes CFS/ME is caused by 'profound disturbances of, and damage to, the neuro-endocrine-immune systems of these patients'. (This is his only explanation for the severity of CFS/ME's symptoms – many sufferers are wheelchair- or bed-bound – in otherwise healthy people. Gulf War Illness (GFI), another of Hooper's specialisms, has clear parallels with CFS/ME. 'Gulf war patients are clearly ill,' Hooper told Burn. 'Fit young men walking on sticks. They have obviously been poisoned, but will anyone do proper tests for the toxins we know they have been exposed to? They will not.')

CFS/ME is a complex, ambiguous illness, and only time will tell if Hooper's theory holds water. Clearly, there's something wrong with these people; yet a report in the *British Medical Journal* in May 2004 confirmed that GPs remained sceptical about CFS/ME, describing sufferers as 'failing to conform to the work ethic' and ignoring 'every effort to get well as quickly as possible', as if getting better was something you just did, like switching on the telly.

Shamefully, GPs have in the past been encouraged in this view by their own magazine, *Pulse*, which advised readers in October 2001: 'Never let the patients know you think ME doesn't exist and is a disease of malingerers... At the end of the consultation, I say goodbye, not au revoir. Always refer ME patients to a local expert. It's a wonderful way of passing the buck.'

SUPPOSED TO BE NICE

It's December 2003 and I am in Los Angeles to interview Gwyneth Paltrow for *Time Out*'s Christmas double issue. An hour before I'm scheduled to meet her – for a drink at a hotel in Beverly Hills – my friend Alice phones from London. Someone she knows at EMI, Coldplay's record label, has tipped her off that Paltrow is pregnant. The reason I've had to risk Deep Vein Thrombosis by flying across the world to meet the actress even though she spends most of her time in London with her husband, Coldplay's Chris Martin, is that she's gone to LA *specifically to announce the pregnancy to the media.*

This is really bad.

'You've got to ask her about it,' says Alice. 'She's going on *Oprah* tomorrow.'

'I can't.'

'You can. In fact, you'll look really stupid if you don't.'

'What if she's offended and walks out?'

'She won't. She's supposed to be nice.'

'But it's invasive of her privacy.'

'For God's sake! She's about to announce it to the world!' She pauses. 'You survived the flight, then.'

'Just about. I was so worried about DVT, I took four aspirin. Now I'm covered in bruises because my blood isn't clotting properly...'

'Better bruised than dead.'

'I suppose,' I say, 'when you put it like that.'

The second I hang up, the back of my left eye begins to throb.

I lie on the hotel bed and will it to stop. The cab to take me to the interview will be here in 15 minutes. What should I do? What can I do?

If I ask Paltrow about her pregnancy and she takes offence, she might cancel the photo shoot planned for the following day – a photo shoot which, like all photo shoots with Hollywood stars, has taken weeks of delicate negotiation to set up. Then we'd have nothing to put on the cover except a crap graphic of a snowflake. (Ironically, the crap graphic of a snowflake sometimes shifts more copies of the magazine than the Hollywood star, but that's another story.)

I have in my washbag a packet containing 24 tablets of the prescription painkiller Kapake. I swallow three for good measure, washing them down with a whisky miniature I forgot to drink on the plane over. There is, I know, a danger that the combination of tablets and alcohol will make me feel drowsy, even nauseous; but if all goes to plan the whisky will calm my nerves while the painkillers work on my head. Result: I will be able to walk, talk and think at the same time.

The drive from West Hollywood where I am staying to Beverly Hills seems to take forever. Every headlight of every passing car brings a fresh sparkle of pain. I want someone to hold an icepack against my forehead; but not as much as I want to sleep, very deeply, for a very long time.

By the time I reach the hotel I'm feeling pretty spacey, and completely fail to appreciate how underdressed I must look in my old jeans and Gap corduroy jacket. In a room off to my left some sort of party is going on. There's a fuzz of chatter, overlaid with tinkling piano. So soothing. I feel submerged, my eyes portholes in the overpressurised U-boat of my head.

When Paltrow appears, bang on time, I shuffle forward like a cartoon sleepwalker and extend a hand. She looks beautiful – a Narnian emissary come to rescue me from this lowly world. White-witchy blonde hair falls about her shoulders, and she has an... aura, that's the only word for it: a compelling aura of serenity.

She shakes my hand. 'Hi,' she says. 'I'm Gwyneth.'

'Hi,' I say. 'I'm John.'

Throbthrobthrob goes my head.

Paltrow decides we will take tea outside. This seems like a good idea, probably because it's hers. Vacantly, I follow her through the sort-of-party room to a sparsely populated patio area. The music and chatter seem very loud.

We order tea. I bring out my cobalt-blue A4 notebook and open it at the questions I compiled on the flight over. In the cramped purgatory of Economy they had at least made sense. Now they seem incomprehensible – random words, floating off the page like butterflies.

Paltrow asks: 'When did you get here?'

'Last night.'

'And how long are you staying?'

'Until tomorrow.'

'What?' she says, apparently surprised. 'You've come all this way...?'

She doesn't finish the sentence, but '...just to meet me' hangs in the air between us.

Of course I bloody have. You're Gwyneth Paltrow.

The tea arrives. I try to pour it, but my hand is shaking so much that most of it goes in the saucer.

'So,' I say, through a fog of pure pain. 'LA seems really nice.'

For a split second, Paltrow looks at me as if my brain has fallen out of my head and on to my lap. Then she goes back to being poised and professional. 'Yeah,' she says, sweetly. 'It's kind of a nice place to visit, see the people you like... and then leave.'

Nodding, I try again to pour my tea. This time, most of it goes in the cup, which is a result. I try to pick the cup up and carry it towards my mouth. Tea sloshes everywhere – all over the table, all over my jeans.

I abort the exercise. Which is fine; except that it involves doing something extraordinary. It involves giving the impression that, having decided to take a sip of tea, I've suddenly, for no particular reason, thought better of it. Mid-sip.

Paltrow looks at me oddly while all this is going on. I hope she doesn't think I'm on drugs. Oh, hang on – I am, after a fashion. One of young Hollywood's favourite recreational drugs, Vicodin, is almost identical in composition to Kapake – codeine with a paracetamol chaser. I imagine the post-interview conversation between the clean-living, macrobiotic Paltrow and her agent:

'*The guy from* Time Out *was kind of wired...*'
'*Rea-lly?*'

'Yeah.'

'Well. We won't be talking to them again.'

Like a robot, I read out my questions in the order I wrote them on the plane. What they relate to, or whether they have any thematic coherence, I have no idea. I might as well be reading out a shopping list. Some sort of mental reflex has kicked in; a lower function come to the rescue of a higher one. As I speak, I steady myself by clutching the underside of the table.

Somewhere in the middle of Paltrow's answer to a particularly po-faced question about whether the film we're there to discuss, a biopic of the poet Sylvia Plath, infringes the privacy of Plath's still-living children, I feel an urgent need to vomit. Not because of any deficiency in her answer, which subsequent appraisal reveals to be measured and sensible, but because the inside of my head is having a full costume run-through for Armageddon.

'Sorry,' I say, getting up. 'Will you excuse me for a minute?'

I make it to the toilet just in time. When I emerge, the cloakroom attendant pointedly looks the other way. Standing at the sink, I wipe the tell-tale traces of vomit from around my mouth. I feel a bit better now.

Miraculously, Paltrow is still there when I get back.

I can't wait any longer. I just need to get this over with. I say: 'There's something I have to ask you.'

'Oh,' she says, looking scared. 'Right.'

'And I feel kind of awkward about it.'

'Okay.'

'And it's that, um, well… I understand that, er, congratulations might be in order?'

There is a silence. A long silence. The sort of silence I like to think astronauts enjoy while observing the Great Wall of China from space.

Then Paltrow smiles beatifically and says: 'Why thank you, yes, they are.'

GREAT BIG FAT FLOATING

By the time I get back to the hotel, the pain has rheostatted up to the point where my head is the only part of my body I can feel – a lolling, hollowed-out pumpkin into which a team of Olympic-standard needle-stabbers is stabbing needles.

The tablets haven't worked. I must have taken them too late: during a migraine attack the stomach seizes up and becomes 'hypotonic', with the result that its contents are unable to reach the small intestine, where they are absorbed into the bloodstream.

I lie on the bed in the darkness and try to visualise what's going on in my brain. A technique called 'biofeedback', this can occasionally cause the migraine to abate. Migraines are the result of a change in blood flow to the brain. Triggers such as stress, particular foods, tobacco smoke or too little/too much sleep cause the arteries at the base of the brain to spasm. This makes them constrict, which reduces the supply of blood to the brain, which causes platelets to clump together, which causes serotonin to be released, which constricts the arteries further, which causes arteries within the brain to dilate so that the brain isn't starved of oxygen. Unsurprisingly, this dilation hurts.

The rational bit of me knows that this is only a migraine; that if I'm able to sleep, even for an hour, it will probably disappear.

But all I can think about are brain tumours.

I think about brain tumours a lot. Great big fat floating brain tumours. It doesn't help that they have such beautifully onomatopoeic names.

Meningioma.

Medulloblastomas.

Haemangioblastomas.

In the 17th century, the disease people feared was bubonic plague. In the 18th century it was syphilis, and in the 19th tuberculosis.

> In 1993, one girl in a suburban American high school infected 400 people with tuberculosis.

Since then it has been cancer, a disease of old age (mostly) whose prevalence may reflect little more than how much longer we all live nowadays.

Cancer comes from the Greek 'karkinos', meaning 'crab'; it shares the creature's uncommon stealth. Cancer is scary because it is always serious and always painful and often fatal. It can also be bafflingly random – though the fact of genetic predisposition means it's more random for some than others. Perhaps temperament also plays a part. In *Illness As Metaphor*, the late Susan Sontag (cancer, since you ask) contrasts the pale, interesting 'tubercular' personality with the 'cancer' personality – antisocial, underexercised, simmering with petty dissatisfactions. Her point is that such thinking is specious and crass, but that can't stop me seeing myself in this definition. It can't stop me wondering if my cynicism is any less of an occupational hazard than squirming nakedly up a chimney flue was for the Victorian urchin-sweeps who went on to develop 'soot warts' on their scrotums.

One in three people develop cancer during their lives; one in four die from it. Between 1971 and 2001, the incidence of cancer increased by around 20 per cent in males and 39 per cent in females. The cancers with the highest five-year relative survival rates are colon cancer (around 47 per cent), cancers of the bladder, cervix and prostate (56-65 per cent) and breast cancer (78 per cent). In the UK in 2002, 3,321 people died as a result of brain tumours – small fry compared to the 33,602 who died of lung cancer, but still…

There's a good chance I've got a brain tumour. Then again, I might have something even worse.

I used to think there wasn't anything worse than a brain tumour. But that was BS (Before Sam).

As I lie on the bed, shivering with pain, ears plugged in a futile attempt to keep out the din of traffic, the story of my old university friend Sam wafts across my brain like poison gas.

SAM'S STORY

About two years ago, Sam was working as a journalist in Washington DC. It wasn't a great time in his life. His girlfriend had just dumped him and his best friend had died of cancer – all in the space of a fortnight. He didn't want to be there. He wanted to be at home in London, eating pies and watching *Footballers' Wives*.

One day, Sam was lunching a contact – an adviser to the US treasury secretary – when he found himself unable to speak. His tongue started palpitating involuntarily. Spasming, you might say. Grabbing a pen, Sam wrote on a paper napkin the words 'Can't talk' and pushed it across the table at his contact. The contact freaked out. He kept standing up, then sitting down;

kept saying 'Oh Jesus' and 'Holy shit'. The contact called to the waiter for water, iced water – now! He was about to call 911 when, gasping, Sam slumped back in his chair and announced, with biblical portentousness, 'It's over.'

Four days later, it happened again. This time the tongue-spasming was accompanied by a migraine-like headache so intense that Sam could relieve the pain only by displacing it – by stabbing himself in the arm with a fork. Terrified, he went to see a doctor. The idea of seeing a US doctor excited him. They were supposed to be good, weren't they? They knew what they were doing, didn't they?

The doctor said, 'Are you stressed? It sounds like stress.' Sam explained that his girlfriend had just dumped him and his best friend had died of cancer. The doctor said, 'It sounds like you're having panic attacks.' He prescribed Sam the anti-anxiety drug Xanax.

Sam loved Xanax. It was so liberating, no longer giving a toss about anything! Even better, the headaches and attacks stopped.

Sam's time in the US came to an end, and he moved back to London. He ate some pies and watched what was left of *Footballers' Wives*. Three days later, he was shopping in Hamleys when he had another attack. It was his worst one yet. He fell to the floor, twitching violently.

Thereafter, he had an average of one attack per day. He went to see his GP, who asked 'Are you stressed?' Sam gave him

101

the girlfriend/best friend speech. The GP said, 'It sounds like you're having panic attacks.' But he also referred him to a neurologist, 'just in case'.

The neurologist gave Sam a cursory physical examination before sending him for a MRI scan. Later that same day, he called Sam and said, 'I need to see you first thing tomorrow morning.'

'Why?' asked Sam.

'There seems to be something in your head,' said the consultant.

Sam arrived at the clinic expecting to be told what it was they'd found. But it transpired that they didn't really know. The radiologist had written on his form: 'Tuberculosis???' The consultant pointed to a dark shadow on the scan. He said he didn't think it was a tumour.

'That's good,' said Sam. 'What is it then?'

'It could be any number of things,' said the consultant.

The consultant put Sam on anti-epilepsy drugs. But it turned out he was allergic to them. He ended up in hospital, on a drip – temperature raging, liver failing. He had blood tests, several spinal taps, more scans.

His consultant tried to console him. 'Look,' he said, 'these things happen. There's something weird in your head, we don't know what it is, but you'll be fine. You can live your life as an epileptic. Plenty of people do. All we have to do is find the right drug for you.'

Sam was starting to get really pissed off with his consultant. But one day, while he was showing Sam some new scans of his brain, another consultant walked past. He paused, looked at the scans and frowned, as if noticing something odd. He gestured to

Top 10 most common travel diseases:

1. **Cholera**
2. **Diarrhoea**
3. **Hepatitis A**
4. **Hepatitis B**
5. **Japanese encephalitis**
6. **Malaria**
7. **Meningococcal disease/ meningitis**
8. **Tetanus**
9. **Typhoid fever**
10. **Yellow fever**

Source: Forbes.com

Sam's consultant to follow him into the corridor.

A few minutes later, both consultants reappeared. The new consultant asked Sam if he'd been to Mexico or India in the last three years. Sam said yes, he'd been to both.

'And did you eat pork while you were there?'

'Yes,' said Sam. 'In Mexico I had some sort of spaghetti bolognaise. It was disgusting. I was with a coach party and we were all sick afterwards.'

'Ah,' said the new consultant. 'What about India?'

'I ate at street stalls in Delhi.'

'Meat?'

'Oh yes,' said Sam, cheerily. 'Lots of meat.'

'Ah,' said the new consultant.

'What's the matter?' asked Sam.

'Well,' said the consultant, 'it seems to me that you've got neurocysticercosis.'

Obviously, Sam had absolutely no idea what this was; so the consultant patiently explained that the strange patches on Sam's MRI scan were cystic lesions. Their presence suggested that a parasite – 'think of it as a worm' – had made a little home for itself inside his brain.

Sam burst into tears.

Actually, cysticercosis is by no means uncommon. Fifty million people around the world suffer from it. It's endemic in Latin America, Africa and Asia, though if you're unlucky you can also pick it up in Portugal, Spain and some Eastern European countries. It's a parasitic infection of the central nervous system caused by the mite *Taenia solium* in its larval stage. Once you've ingested the parasite, usually by eating bad pork, it migrates through your body and can end up anywhere – your ankle, your knee, your lungs, your heart. (It only becomes neurocysticercosis if and when it enters your brain.)

That Sam was still alive was, his new consultant declared, a miracle. Since then he has responded well to treatment. The parasite has calcified and will trouble him no more.

Understandably, it's taken Sam a long time to accept this.

He'd always been quite a hardy, risk-taking sort of person. Now, every time he gets a cold he thinks he's dying. Even when his treatment had technically finished, he took to pestering his consultant with visits and questions until one day the guy snapped.

'Look, Sam,' he said. 'I spend my whole life hacking into people's brains. And you have to understand this: practically no-one I touch gets better. If they do, it's because I've lobotomised them. Neurology is the most depressing area of medicine. You're the one person in the last ten years who's been cured – cured because I was able to spot what was wrong with you and treat you effectively. Now go away, and I hope I never see you again.'

WHAT DOES IT ALL MEAN?

Over the last hundred years, the brain has replaced the digestive system as the prime focus of hypochondriac anxiety. Even people who would never describe themselves as hypochondriacs imagine great blossoming brain tumours whenever they get a severe headache. (I imagine a particular type of tumour – a butterfly glioma, which drapes itself across the brain, a wing on each hemisphere.)

Others, like the American poet Sara Teasdale, fear strokes. Teasdale, stiflingly overprotected as a child, spent much of the rest of her life cloistered like an invalid. When, in January 1933, a small blood vessel in her hand ruptured, she inter-preted it as a sign that she was about to suffer a massive cerebral haemorrhage and killed herself with an overdose of sleeping pills.

(She foretold this act in a mournful, Emily Dickinsonian poem from her collection *In a Hospital*:

'Great Sower when you tread
My field again
Scatter the furrows there
With better grain.')

Hypochondria is only partly about the sensation of pain or discomfort; it's about what that pain or discomfort might mean. As Fugen Neziroglu explains in the July 1998 issue of *Psychiatric Times*: 'The hypochondriacal patient seems more concerned with the authenticity, meaning or etiological significance of symptoms rather than with unpleasant physical sensations.'

You can see why the brain would be the focus of such overinterpretation. After all, the brain is different. If you get gangrene in your foot, you can get that foot chopped off. It won't be a pleasant experience, but chances are you'll still be the same person when the anaesthetic wears off. The foot is not the theatre of consciousness. It is not the seat of the soul.

Not that I believe in such a thing as a soul. I know from reading neuropsychologist Paul Brok's terrifying, brilliant *Into the Silent Land* that to speak of a unified self is hopeful, quasi-mystical nonsense:

'From a neuroscience perspective we are all divided and discontinuous. The mental processes underlying our sense of self – feelings, thoughts, memories – are scattered through different zones of the brain. There is no special point of convergence. No cockpit of the soul. No soul pilot.'

In other words, there is no part of your brain you can injure and be absolutely sure it isn't going to affect your fundamental sense of who you are. This is why I am terrified of something going wrong with my brain; why I am terrified of Alzheimer's and its affiliated genres of senility. (In one of the most disturbing types of dementia, Cotard's syndrome or 'le délire de negation', patients cease to believe that they exist. Though actually, I often feel like this at 5pm on a Friday afternoon.)

I have on video somewhere a documentary about John F Kennedy's assassination which shows most of the famous Zapruder footage of the shooting and its grisly aftermath. You can see, quite clearly, Kennedy's head splitting apart and a bit of his brain falling out. I can't watch it without bringing a hand up to touch the back of my head, to keep my brain in place.

But I can't keep my brain in place. I can't stop it from worrying about itself.

MIDNIGHT-ISH

Unlike Sam, I don't want to see an American doctor. I'm worried on two counts:

1. They'll find something wrong which a British doctor, with his/her endearingly no-nonsense pragmatism and antiquated equipment, wouldn't find.

2. They'll send me a bill for $25,000 for a half-hour appointment and my travel insurance won't cover it and we'll have to sell the house.

Luckily, I feel a lot better after a few hours' sleep. I look at my alarm clock. It's midnight-ish. This means I can phone Cathy in London, where it's 8am-ish.

'Hello,' I say.

'Oh, hi. How did it go?'

'I had a migraine.'

'Again? You should see someone. That's your third in just over a week.' Cathy sounds uncharacteristically concerned. 'Did you have to cancel the interview?'

'I struggled through like the trouper I am.'

'You did?' She sounds surprised. 'Well, it can't have been that bad. But you should still go and see Gimpface. Tell him you want to be referred to someone.'

I ask the question even though I know what the answer will be. 'Do you think I've got a brain tumour?'

'No. Stop being ridiculous.'

Back in London, I make another appointment to see Gimpface. He has a black eye. Before I get the chance to ask if this was inflicted by an enraged patient he explains: 'Rugby accident.'

'Ah,' I nod, feeling even more than usual like a girl.

HE REFERRED ME

I can't believe it. Gimpface referred me. This means he thinks there's a good chance I have a brain tumour. And if *he* thinks I have a brain tumour, I must have one.

Hang on, though – that doesn't follow. He's always been hopeless in the past. Why assume some revolution in his diagnostic capacity just because it tallies with my own suspicions?

To take what remains of my mind off all this, I settle down

to read Dr F Clifford Rose and Dr M Gawel's book, *Migraine: The Facts*, a recent second-hand purchase. It's quite an eye-opener, and I feel vaguely ashamed by how ordinary my migraines are when some people's seem to resemble Pink Floyd concerts:

'The whole visual field may be fragmented and interrupted by shiny lines, arranged like constellations, a phenomenon known as fortification spectra, because of its resemblance to a castellated fort. (Some mystics have interpreted these as visions of "the eternal city".)'

Fortification Spectra! Now that's a great name for a band. Much better than Cancer Cluster.

> **Four different phrases for cancer:**
> Opacification
> Mass
> Neoplastic involvement
> Mitotic process

The doctors continue: 'There may also be small multicoloured areas of flashing lights, zigzag patterns, or "Catherine Wheels", and there is usually generalised blurring of vision, as if looking through steam or water.'

There is a chapter on headaches which aren't migraine but might be serious all the same. Apart from the bit about 'ice-cream headaches' ('caused by holding very cold substances in the mouth'), this chapter isn't so entertaining.

'Patients with cerebral haemorrhage nearly always have a headache,' I read, 'particularly if the blood gets into the space surrounding the brain (sub-arachnoid haemorrhage). This bleeding often arises from a weakened part of a blood vessel which has ballooned out forming an aneurysm, or occasionally from an abnormal congenital group of blood vessels – an angioma.'

I look up, worried. Angioma. That 'ang'... It sounds a bit like... telangiectasias!

And what was it the *Medline Plus Medical Encyclopedia* said? Telangiectasias may also occur in the brain.

That must be what my headaches are! Maybe the bleeding has, until now, been so slow as to be imperceptible but has suddenly reached a critical stage.

Shit.

I must mention it to the consultant next week. If I'm still alive by then.

SOLID AUTHORITY

With its jaunty blue colour scheme and lack of visible medical apparatus, Dr _____'s office is more like a sitting room than a doctor's surgery. A huge cushion-strewn sofa runs the entire length of one wall. As I enter, Dr _____ rises from behind an oak desk wedged into the far corner and shakes my hand in a manly fashion.

'Sit down,' he barks softly.

I sit down. Dr _____ clearly dislikes small talk, a tic I interpret as efficiency rather than a desire to bundle me out of the room as quickly as possible. Private health insurance being a recently acquired luxury, I have never visited a clinic like this before. Already I feel soothed by how comfortable the room is, and by the atmosphere of solid authority it exudes.

'So,' says Dr _____. 'When did you last have a migraine?'

'Last week. I was in Los Angeles for work.'

'What do you do?'

'I'm a journalist.'

'Ah.' He nods. 'A high migraine risk category.'

I tell Dr _____ about my headaches. He listens, takes notes, nods. When I've finished, he beckons me towards a proper Freudian-style couch I hadn't noticed before. As I lie on it, arms by my side like a tin soldier, Dr _____ hovers above me, whispering random words and waving his hands around. It's quite some pantomime.

Afterwards, I ask: 'What were you doing?'

'Testing your reflexes,' says Dr _____.

Now seems a good time to tax him with my straight-to-the-point questions.

Clearing my throat, I ask, 'Have I got a worm in my brain?'

'A worm?'

'Neurocysticercosis. A friend of mine had it. He got it in India, or maybe Mexico.'

Dr _____ narrows his eyes. 'And what makes you think you've got it too?'

'One of his symptoms was headaches.'

Dr _____ scratches the back of his neck. He stares blankly at the wall behind my head. All of a sudden the atmosphere of comfort shrivels in the glare of a greater truth: I am terrified of this man. But I must ask him my second question or I'll hate myself afterwards.

'Assuming the answer to that last question is no…'

'A safe assumption.'

'…what about telangiectasias?'

'What about it?'

'I've got a spot. On my chest. It's a vascular lesion. And I read somewhere that you can get them in your brain.'

'It's possible.' Dr _____ pauses. 'Where did you say you read that?'

'I didn't.'

'Was it on the internet?'

'I can't remember.'

'Who identified the spot on your chest as a vascular lesion?'

'Gimpface.'

Whoops!

'Who?'

'My doctor. He likes to be called... It's an affectionate, um... We play rugby together.'

Dr _____ and I are staring at each other. With my stare I am trying to communicate that I will not be discouraged or browbeaten. With his stare he is trying to communicate that I am at best a toad, possibly a weasel.

He breaks the silence. 'My diagnosis is that you're suffering from common migraine. I'm going to prescribe you some anti-inflammatory wafers which you should dissolve under your tongue when you feel an attack coming on. They're expensive but they work really well.'

'Great. Thank you.'

'So I think that's it.'

'Good.'

'Apart from the MRI scan.'

The shock is clearly visible on my face.

'Oh yes,' he says. 'It's always good to be sure.'

JIM FIXED IT FOR ME

Down, down I go, into the bowels of the building. In a wooden cubicle I remove my clothes and slip on a paper gown. The radiologist wafts over and asks if I've ever had a scan before. Her voice is breezily neutral – she might be welcoming me to a Harvester restaurant. I shake my head. She tells me that magnetic resonance imaging works by using a strong magnetic field to scan hydrogen protons in the body.

She asks me if I'm wearing eye make-up.

'No,' I say. 'Why?'

She explains that it can degrade the quality of the image.

Do I look like I'm wearing eye make-up? It's always good to have new things to worry about.

The woman leads me over to a padded plastic cradle and hands me a pair of headphones to keep out the thumpthumpthump-gragragra-nnhnnhnnh. The cradle is comfier than it looks, and as it slides slowly into the tunnel

The age-standardised rate for deaths involving MRSA in males increased from 14.8 per million population in 2002 to 16.3 per million in 2003.
In females the rate increased from 7.0 to 8.5 per million population over the same perod.

– the throbbing, elongated heart of the magnet – I get a sudden flashback of all the *Blue Peter* bring-and-buy sales I took part in as a child, all the scanners my fellow *Blue Peter* viewers and I helped to buy for all those children's hospitals... And now here I am in one! Even with the headphones on the thumpthumpthump-gragragra-nnhnnhnnh is deafening. I wonder if Cornish techno wizard the Aphex Twin ever had a MRI scan as a child. If so, maybe he was visited in hospital afterwards by the veteran DJ and fixer of things for children, Jimmy Saville? It would account for a lot.

'So,' I ask the radiologist as I'm clambering off the cradle half an hour later, 'were there any suspicious black patches?'

She smiles thinly. 'I can't tell you that. You'll have to make an appointment to see Dr _____ again next week.'

'Oh go on. Give me a clue.'

'No.'

'Just answer me this. Is it worth our while booking a summer holiday?'

PHILIP LARKIN'S OESOPHAGUS

Fear of illness is not just fear of illness. It is a fear of incapacity, dependency, pain, immobility, hospitals and death, and the greatest of these is death. Hypochondriacs don't, on the whole, suspect themselves of having the sort of illnesses that a few dosed-up days in bed could cure. They fear big diseases, serious diseases – diseases you can die from.

On March 16 1985, the poet Philip Larkin went to see a cardiologist at Hull Nuffield Hospital. Larkin had always worried about his health, but it had started to deteriorate more noticeably. The usual symptoms of his usual complaints – piles, constipation, sleeplessness – had been augmented by what Larkin called 'cardio-spasms'. In Larkin's medical notes, the cardiologist noted that Larkin was suffering from depression and hypochondria. He had, he wrote, 'a cancer phobia and fear of dying'.

Already, on March 7, Larkin had had a barium meal after complaining of difficulty swallowing. He wrote to his friend Judy Egerton, apologising for not having contacted her for ages and giving as an excuse the fact that he was 'in a sort of flap' about his health, which had 'occasioned various excursions into the world of X-rays and blood tests'. Larkin had always had difficulties with his oesophagus. Before each meal, he would drink a huge glass of water to force it open. Tests soon revealed it to be the source of his problems: he had a polypoid tumour on it which would require surgery.

Larkin was obsessed by the idea that he would die at the same age as his father, 63. In a review of DJ Enright's *Oxford Book of Death*, published in 1983, he wrote: 'Man's most remarkable talent is for ignoring death. For once the certainty of permanent extinction is realised, only a more immediate calamity can dislodge it from the mind, and then only temporarily.'

The operation to remove Larkin's oesophagus revealed widespread cancer, not just in the oesophagus but in his throat, which was too advanced to be removable by surgery.

His girlfriend Monica decided to spare Larkin the full force of this information. But Larkin knew the end was near. He shut himself away, drank only cheap red wine and ate only Complan.

He died at 1.24am on Monday, December 2. His last words, uttered to the nurse who was gripping his hand, were: 'I am going to the inevitable.'

Larkin, of course, wrote the best ever poem about fear of death, 'Aubade'. It was one of his final poems. Published in 1977, it had taken him three years to write.

'I work all day, and get half drunk at night.
Waking at four to soundless dark, I stare.
In time the curtain-edges will grow light.
Till then I see what's really always there:
Unresting death, a whole day nearer now,
Making all thought impossible but how
And where and when I shall myself die.
Arid interrogation: yet the dread
Of dying, and being dead,
Flashes afresh to hold and horrify.'

People's opinion of 'Aubade' seems to hinge on how convincing they find the line about 'the dread/ Of dying, and being dead'. It works for me. It didn't for Larkin's friend

118

Kingsley Amis, whose critique of the poem in his *Memoirs* is memorably no-nonsense:

> 'If you can't think you can't realise you haven't any senses and aren't anywhere, and don't tell me again it'll be different from before you were born because (though you had nothing to think with then either) you could pass the time by looking forward to your birth. I know the paths of glory and everything else lead but to the grave. And on first reading "Aubade", I should have found a way of telling you that depression among the middle-aged and elderly is common in the early morning and activity disperses it, so if you feel as bad as you say then fucking get up, or if it's too early or something then put the light on and read Dick Francis.'

HOW COME YOU'RE STILL ALIVE?

The death of a friend or parent is one of the most common triggers of hypochondria. One chronic sufferer, Nick, links his to his father's death at 64, just over ten years ago.

'I went through a phase,' he says, 'of thinking that because he had died aged 64 and I was approaching 32, I was halfway through my own life. It seemed perfectly reasonable for me to assume that his life was a template for my own. A year after he died I found myself getting increasingly worked up about this. I'd pass men in the street who looked older than 64 and think: You bastard. How come you're alive? What makes you so special?

'Grief counselling helped with this to some degree, but I still have an all-consuming fear of contracting a terminal illness before I've reached an acceptable age to die. And as I'm 41 now, and I've always regarded 50 as middle age, that age for me is 100.

'My father was a hypochondriac, though he hid from us the full extent of it. He was always managing to convince himself that he had cancer in whichever part of his body he had some symptom he could interpret that way; always going to his GP, who kept fobbing him off. The thing is, of course, that in the end he was proved right – he had lymphoma, which killed him. He didn't catch it early enough, and if he had he might have been cured.

'So the big scare for me is never, say, heart disease – it's always cancer. Whenever I have a lump anywhere I think it's cancer, though so far it's always been explained away as a sebaceous cyst or an inflamed hair follicle.'

In 'Aubade', Larkin denounces as 'specious stuff' the view that 'no rational being can fear a thing it will not feel'. This is right and proper. How, after all, do you know that you won't feel death?

I expect to feel mine, and my layman's knowledge of cancer

suggests to me that I will, intensely, especially at those points when my morphine drip stops working.

WOMEN AND MEN

We are sitting having dinner: me, Cathy, Cathy's friend Miriam and Miriam's partner, Ben. I have cooked a beef casserole based on an Elizabethan recipe from a National Trust cookbook. It's heavy on prunes, ale and cloves. It's supposed to be made with lamb, but they didn't have any lamb in Sainsbury's so I had to get beef. I'm a bit nervous about eating beef – I haven't eaten it at all since the start of the BSE scare, even organic beef – but increasingly I feel it's a hang-up I should, well, hang up. I can't spend the rest of my life not eating beef on spurious health grounds.

I decide to say out loud, to everyone at the table: 'In case you're wondering why I've suddenly started eating beef, it's because I've decided I can't spend the rest of my life not eating it on spurious health grounds.'

'I didn't know you had *stopped* eating beef,' says Miriam, who likes to crush epiphanies underfoot.

But Ben says: 'I know what John means. I had a similar thing the other month. When there was all that fuss about the chilli powder with that Sudan 1 dye in it? I stopped eating readymeals, sausages, salad dressing. And then I thought: This is rubbish. Think of the tiny quantity of Sudan 1 that must be present in the amount of Worcester Sauce they'd add to a shepherd's pie. It's not going to kill you, is it? It's not like that's going to kill you and a diet of crisps and Diet Coke isn't. Half the children I teach eat nothing else but crisps and Diet Coke.'

'You know,' says Miriam, 'if I actually thought you believed that, I'd be really impressed.'

Ben folds his arms. 'I do believe it.'

'When the dye thing was in the news every day,' Miriam explains, 'Ben got so worried he went to see our GP. He'd eaten one of the dodgy Marks & Spencer Steam Cuisine chicken things. He had this pain below his stomach. He was going on and on about it. He said he thought the dye had accumulated in his kidneys and they were about to fail.'

Cathy and Miriam laugh uproariously. Ben and I don't.

***

Are men bigger hypochondriacs than women? Women are supposedly better at reporting symptoms to doctors than men. They go to the doctor more. A 1999 survey of health service use found that in 1998-99, in both the 16 to 24 and the 25 to 34 age groups, half as many men as women consulted an NHS GP in the previous two weeks. In his book *The Psychopathology of Women*, Ihsan Al-Issa wonders if this isn't because 'the expression of malaise and distress by women is more acceptable because these complaints overlap with culturally learned patterns of normal female behaviour'. (Though how many of these women would have been seeing their GPs about pregnancy – or child-related issues? Is it really a surprise that women, their bodies contorted by the force of another human being growing inside them, might worry about their health more than men?)

A WOMAN: AUNT ETTY

Henrietta, or 'Aunt Etty' as she was known to her niece Gwen Raverat, was Emma and Charles Darwin's second daughter. Throughout her life, as Raverat's autobiography *Period Piece* reveals, Etty followed her father's example, setting herself up as a sort of invalid supreme; yet no one could remember what was supposed to be wrong with her. At the age of 15 she'd been ordered by the doctor to have breakfast in bed – so she insisted on having breakfast in bed every day for the rest of her life. Raverat writes that Etty was 'always going away to rest in case she might be tired later on in the day, or even the next day. She would send down to the cook to ask her to count the prune-stones left on her plate, as it was very important to know whether she had eaten three or four prunes for luncheon.'

She was terrified of colds. Whenever anyone in the house had a cold she took to bed wearing a home-made gas-mask device. This was 'an ordinary wire kitchen-strainer, stuffed with antiseptic cotton-wool, and tied on like a snout with elastic over her ears'. Etty felt a close kinship with Mr Woodhouse from *Emma*. She had the same almost professional interest in other people's health. Says Raverat: 'There was a kind of sympathetic gloating in the Darwin voices, when they said, for instance, to one of us children: "And have you got a *bad* sore throat, my poor cat?"... It was exactly the voice in which Mr Woodhouse must have spoken of "Poor Miss Taylor".'

A MAN: SAMUEL PEPYS

And yet, and yet... Some men have an almost autistic ability not to notice disease. Samuel Pepys made it through 1665 barely conscious that, all around him, people were dropping dead from bubonic plague. The common cold, though – *that* bothered him. February 1665 was very cold – Europe was in the grip of a mini-Ice Age – and at one point in his diaries he worries that he might be coming down with an ague on account of having worn an insufficiently aired coat.

The big discussion all middle-class London families were

having was whether or not to leave the city. (Daniel Defoe's *Journal of the Plague Year* opens with two brothers arguing about this.) By June 1665, it's obvious things are bad. Pepys's own doctor, Alexander Burnet, shuts up his house for the stipulated forty-day quarantine period because one of his servants has got it. This is a significant event – it proves that the plague isn't just a disease of poor households.

Yet Pepys carries on as normal, buying stockings at the Royal Exchange and books at St Paul's and visiting his bankers. He even makes a totally needless journey to a plague pit in Moorfields, just to satisfy his morbid curiosity. He has a scare in a hackney coach when the driver has to stop because he's 'suddenly stroke very sick and almost blind', but it doesn't worry him too much. There are more important things on his mind – mistresses like linen draper Betty Martin, with whom he does 'what he voudrais… both devante and backward'.

Only in August does he leave town. He boasts in a letter of having 'stayed in the city till about 7400 died in one week, and of them above 6000 of the plague, and little noise heard day nor night but tolling of bells'. The truth is, he is enjoying himself so much that the plague simply doesn't impinge on his life. He's been given two new appointments – treasurer to the Tangier Committee and surveyor-general of victualling for the navy. He's been elected to the Royal Society. His personal fortune has quadrupled. He wrote: 'I have never lived so merrily (besides that I never got so much) as I have done this plague-time.'

SELL-BY DATES

1993. I am driving along the M6 with my girlfriend, Rachel, listening to 'So Tough' by Saint Etienne. Actually, Rachel is driving – driving and smoking. I am in the passenger seat with a box of cassette tapes on my lap. I am Custodian Of The Tapes. I am also Custodian Of The Cigarettes. This means that whenever Rachel clicks her fingers, I place a lit Camel in her mouth, taking care to rip the filter off first.

Rachel eschews filters. She usually smokes French cigarettes which don't have filters, but she's run out, and of the lesser brands available at the last service station we stopped at she would touch only Camels. I don't like it, this filterless smoking, but Rachel thinks it's daring and bohemian – sort of *Betty Blue* but minus the gouged-out eyes.

'Think of all that shit going into your lungs,' I say.

'You eat meat,' she says. 'That's full of shit. We're all putting shit into our bodies all the time.'

'Don't you want to limit it, though? The shit?'

She shrugs. 'Smoking tastes better without a filter.'

(I don't tell her about the time a man from the anti-smoking group ASH came to my school to give a talk. He

126

brought along a tar-ridden human lung in a jar. It slipped from his hands as he was showing it off to us and smashed all over the floor – a shiny, wobbling, stinking mound, less dead-seeming than it should have been. There was screaming, fainting, possibly urination.)

We are on our way to the Lake District, where Rachel's parents have a holiday home. Her father is a doctor. He smokes even more than she does. The whole family smoke. Last time we came here I thought I saw the dog smoking, but I was mistaken – it was standing in front of a barbecue chewing a twig and I was drunk.

I say to Rachel: 'Your dad scares me.'

I say to Rachel: 'I don't think he likes me.'

Rachel says: 'He's a sweetie. You just have to follow his rules.'

'Like what?'

'Well, you know – he likes routine. He likes a glass of sherry in the evening.'

'I can cope with that.'

'He likes his nibbles too. He always makes up a big plate of hors d'oeuvres. Little squares of toast spread with paté with a caper on top.'

'I don't like capers.'

'Pretend.'

'I like paté.'

'Well, the thing about the paté is... It, um... It's just possible that it might have been knocking around slightly longer than the stipulated four days after opening.'

Rachel is telling me this because I told her a few months back about school. About the uncooked sausages and the not-so-purified water. I explained that this was the source of my phobia of eating food past its sell-by date.

Later that evening we are sat in the sitting room, napkins on knee. When it's my turn to take a biscuit from the plate I hesitate. Then my hand does a little shaky dance, as if casting a spell.

'So Dad,' says Rachel. 'How old's this paté? Reassure John.'

'Bought this very morning,' says Mr Winter. He is a large man, dressed down in neatly pressed jeans and brown brogues.

'Really?'

'Absolutely. Though even if it was a week old, it wouldn't do you any harm. It's been in the fridge. And it's packed full of preservatives. Sulphites, probably, with a broad spectrum antimicrobial action.'

In a small quiet voice I say, 'What about its sell-by date?'

There is a silence. Then Rachel's father says, 'I'm sorry?'

'Its sell-by date,' I repeat.

'Do you really think,' Mr Winter booms, 'that there's a precise, objectively determined point at which an open pack of bacon becomes inedible? Or that supermarkets are doing anything more public-spirited than covering their capacious bottoms when they tell you that a wedge of stilton – stilton! – bought on June 21st needs to be consumed by June 29th?'

'I suppose not,' I say. Then I think of something. 'What if I'm allergic to sulphites?'

Mr Winter's eyes bulge dangerously. 'Are you allergic to sulphites?'

'I don't know. But what if I was?'

'There might be an adverse reaction,' he concedes. 'But actually the pathophysiology of sulphite sensitivity isn't as clear as some scientists would have us believe.'

'Dad's maxim is "blind 'em with science",' says Rachel, smiling indulgently.

'If only I could,' he says, 'the silly fuckers.'

I ask him how long he's been a doctor.

He scratches the side of his head. 'Fucked if I can remember. How long's a priest's cock?'

'I don't know,' I say. 'I've only ever seen one.'

I explain that when I was young I always wanted to be a doctor - indeed, that my family nurtured certain expectations of my following in my grandfather's footsteps; that there was a barometer with my name inscribed on it which had been my grandfather's who was also called John O'Connell, blah blah – but was always rubbish at maths and science. 'I think,' I say, 'that I might be numerically dyslexic.'

'Ah yes,' says Mr Winter. 'The traditional fop's defence.'

We chat awkwardly for a few minutes more, then he says: 'Now look, are you going to have one of these biscuits or not?'

What else can I do?

We sleep in bunk beds – me on top, ha ha. Are they comfortable? They are not. To make matters worse, my stomach is emitting troubling squeaks and gurgles.

I call down to Rachel: 'It feels like it's readying itself for something.'

'Sleep?' she asks, hopefully.

'No,' I say. 'It's like it's vacuum-sealing itself – as if it's trying to stop the evil things inside it seeping out into the rest of my body.'

At around 3am I wake up knowing for certain that I am going to be sick. I make it to the bathroom just in time. When the worst of the retching has subsided, I tilt my head to see that Rachel and her family have all shuffled out on to the landing, dressing gowns agape.

The next day there is a walk planned. A walk across five miles of open moorland. A walk through - among many, many other things – fields containing sheep. I explain that I can't possibly go: the risk of contracting Lyme disease, a bacterial infection caused by the bite of infected sheep and deer ticks, is too great.

No one contradicts me.

Hypochondria raises intriguing questions about what it means to be sick or well. If I declare myself to be sick, does that mean I am sick? Is the desire to be sick itself an illness? (Why would anyone want to be sick? Isn't sickness debilitating and inconvenient?)

The fact is, even if I'm convinced I'm sick, I'm not properly sick until I have been pronounced sick by a doctor – until I have been given permission to adopt what the sociologist Talcott Parsons has called 'the sick role'.

The sick role is a mass of competing obligations and privileges. There are three principal obligations:

1. The patient must recognise that the state of being ill is undesirable.
2. He or she must accept an obligation to co-operate with others in order to regain 'health'.
3. He or she must utilise the services of those regarded by society as competent to diagnose and treat illness.

In return, three privileges are granted:

1. An acknowledgement that the patient is not responsible for the state he or she is in.

2. An acceptance of the fact that he or she requires care.

3. A recognition that he or she is exempt from normal social and professional obligations for the duration of the illness.

In very severe hypochondria, where refusal to accept reassurance is held to be evidence of psychotic disorder, doctors will grant permission to adopt the sick role on the condition that the sufferer agrees to be treated. But in mid-spectrum hypochondria, a doctor's refusal to grant this permission in the face of the patient's certainty that it is appropriate is a key source of tension.

In a climate of escalating healthcare costs, the mid-spectrum hypochondriac is nothing less than an enemy of the state. Some of the time, he knows this. He might even try to assuage his guilt by pointing out that history has often judged doctors just as harshly. 'The Arrogance of Physicians in general, and the great Knowledge which they are obliged to pretend to are deservedly Censur'd and Ridiculed by all Men of Sence,' wrote Bernard de Mandeville in *A Treatise of the Hypochondriack and Hysterick Passions* (1711).

Molière's final play, *La malade imaginaire* (1673), mocks as typical a would-be doctor whose wonderfully bullshitty answer to the question 'Why does opium cause sleep?' – 'Because there is in it a dormitive virtue, the nature of which is to sedate the senses' – wins him a round of applause from the body of elders whose job it is to confer medical degrees.

In the original production, the part of the satire's hypochondriacal hero, Argan, was acted by Molière himself. On February 17, 1673, the evening of the play's fourth performance, Molière experienced a severe coughing fit on stage. He struggled back to his apartment, where later that night he suffered a fatal haemorrhage, attended only by some nuns who, for reasons obscure, happened to be lodging with him at the time. Molière's life had been blighted by lung problems, and *Le malade imaginaire* represents a final explosion of contempt for all the doctors who had so blunderingly failed to cure him. Argan's brother Béralde gets a telling line in the play: 'Medicine is only for those who are fit enough to survive the treatment as well as the illness.'

Total adult per capita alcohol consumption in the UK in 1961 (litres): 6.56
Total adult per capita alcohol consumption in the UK in 1999 (litres): 9.73

Paradoxically, Argon needs the routines prescribed by his doctors to remain well – a phenomenon known as 'iatrogenic' (or 'doctor-reinforced) hypochondria. Doctors have always done very well out of this. In her book *Hypochondria: Woeful Imaginings*, Susan Baur quotes John Moore in his *Medical*

Sketches (1786) estimating that his colleagues received five-sixths of their income from treating 'imaginary complaints, or such as would have disappeared fully as soon as they had been left to themselves. But this ought not to be imputed as a crime to the physician; if an old lady cannot dine with comfort till he has felt her pulse, looked at her tongue, and told her whether her chicken should be roasted or boiled, it is reasonable he should be paid for his trouble.'

The limitations of pre-scientific medicine meant that until the early twentieth century doctors were rarely able to fulfil more than a basic placebo role. Their job was to hold the patient's hand and enact the old familiar rituals. Much of their time was spent comforting victims of fevers like the 'putrid fever' which floors neurasthenic Marianne Dashwood in Jane Austen's *Sense and Sensibility*.

When summoned out on a call, doctors would be welcomed into the home as a cross between a friend and a servant. They would take the patient's history; ask about eating, sleeping and bowel habits; feel the pulse; and listen, without the benefit of a stethoscope, to the chest. And that, really, was that. Decorum prohibited any sort of detailed physical examination: only after Queen Victoria's death did her physician, Sir James Reid, discover that she had a 'ventral hernia, and a prolapse of the uterus'.

Many well-to-do Victorians embraced the sick role

whole-heartedly. Since the majority of middle-class people recovered from illnesses at home, hospitals being largely receptacles for the dying poor, it made sense to hire a nurse and designate a special room – the sick room – in which to house the invalid. Healthcare manuals of the time are heavy on exacting specifications. 'The sick-room furniture ought to have as little drapery as is consistent with neatness,' instructs Esther Le Hardy in *The Home Nurse and Manual for the Sick Room* (1865). 'People coming into the sick room should particularly avoid sitting on the side of the bed, as it tightens the bedclothes and irritates the patient.' Another advises that 'knick-knacks and fine furniture are there sadly out of place, not only on account of the time they waste and the dust and disease they harbour, but on account of *the air they displace* [my italics]'.

Not that a nurse could do very much. Dr R H Bakewell suggests that his readers 'always, unless in a case of sudden illness, send for a medical man early in the day'.

A favourite maxim was: If in doubt, bleed. Bloodletting worked on the baseless assumption that purging the body of its vital life force was the same as purging it of illness. It was called venesection or phlebotomy when it involved opening veins with a knife; but you could also use leeches.

The favoured type was *hirudo medicinalis*. It's one and a half inches long, but expands to six when its stomachs (it has ten) are full. It has both male and female sex organs, and a semicircular mouth with three cartilaginous teeth. Leeches were taken from water an hour before use to give them time to grow hungry. They would then be placed in a wine glass which was upturned on to the patient's body. After 50 minutes they would drop off, full and (generally) asleep. To make them disgorge the blood you sprinkled them with salt. Then you could use them again.

In the pre-scientific era, many people self-diagnosed, dosing themselves with folk cures like savin, juniper and pennyroyal. They sought refuge in religion or magic. The touch of a hanged man's hand was said to cure a multitude of ailments. A stye would vanish if you stroked it with the tail of a black cat. Where these remedies were plant-based, they often worked.

William Withering, a Stafford GP who was also a botanist and the author of the bestselling *A Botanical Arrangement of All Vegetables Naturally Growing in Great Britain*, was riding through rural Shropshire in 1775 when he met an old woman who seemed to be able to cure dropsy – water-retention – with foxglove. The active ingredient in foxglove, the heart stimulant digitalis, entered the *Edinburgh Pharmacopoeia* in 1783. Philosopher Thomas Hobbes declared: 'I would rather have the advice or take physick from an experienced old woman that had been at many sick people's bedsides than from the learnedest but unexperienced physician.'

(Gwen Raverat remembers that, as late as 1947, 'a fried mouse was most earnestly recommended to me as a cure for whooping cough. I dare say it is as good as any other cure; the only difficulty is to believe in it.')

Reading domestic manuals from the eighteenth and nineteenth centuries, you frequently get the impression that the writers are making it up as they go along. On the subject of dealing with scalds and burns, *A Manual of Domestic Economy with Hints on Domestic Medicine and Surgery* (1871) advises that 'another application of great value, which has at the same time the recommendation of being always at hand, and of requiring no skill in its use, is flour':

> 'This should be dusted on thickly with a dredger, so as to
> absorb the discharge, and cover the injured part completely…
> A crust is thus formed which cracks and permits the escape of
> the discharge, and, as the burn heals, it drops off piecemeal.
> This simple remedy is one of the most successful, and is
> adopted in several of the London Hospitals.'

Since Marianne Dashwood's melodramatic near-death from what the advent of sulpha drugs and then penicillin transformed into a non-disease, global life expectancy has more than doubled. In the 50 years since the founding of the

NHS in 1948, infant mortality in England and Wales fell from 39 to 7 in every 1,000 for girls and from 30 to 5 for boys. In the UK, life expectancy has increased from 66 to 74.5 for men, and from 70.5 to just under 80 for women. Between 1971 and 1991, deaths from stroke dropped by 40 per cent and from coronary heart disease by 19 per cent.

This is clearly cause for celebration. So why, then, are we more worried than ever about our health? Was Roy Porter right that 'doctors and "consumers" are becoming locked in a fantasy that everyone has something wrong with them, everyone and everything can be cured'? Have our expectations of medicine grown unreasonably high? Where did it come from, our sense of entitlement to a cure? After all, the Hippocratic Oath doesn't say anything about curing. It starts: 'First, do no harm...'

Scientific medicine is the reason most of us are still alive. And yet many of us are perversely dissatisfied with it. As we trudge into the local health centre, there to see one of five or six time-pressured, bored-seeming GPs who may or may not know us or anything about our medical histories beyond what is scrawled in our notes, it's easy to idealise the pre-scientific past; to feel that the famous American medical professor FW Peabody had a point when he wrote in 1927, at the start of the scientific revolution, that 'young graduates have been taught a great deal about the mechanism of disease, but very little about the practice of medicine – or, to put it more bluntly, they are too "scientific" and do not know how to take care of patients.'

It's certainly the case that the old *Dr Finlay's Casebook*-style doctor no longer exists. In 2003/4, 86 per cent of consultations with NHS GPs in the UK took place in GPs' surgeries. More were conducted over the phone (10 per cent) than in the patient's home (4 per cent). This is a drop of four-fifths since 1971, when 22 per cent of doctors made home visits.

(One of the qualities the serial killer Harold Shipman's patients admired in him was his willingness to treat patients in their own homes. Christopher Rudolf, the son of one of Shipman's victims, was quoted in P Barkham's 'The Shipman Report' in the *Times* on July 20, 2002, as saying: 'I remember the time Dr Shipman gave to my Dad. He would come round at the drop of a hat. He was a marvellous GP.')

Peabody famously declared that 'the practice of medicine in its broadest sense includes the whole relationship of the physician with his patient'. He was particularly interested in 'patients who have "nothing the matter with them"', that 'large group of patients who do not show objective pathologic conditions'. If it's true that, as Peabody says, it is 'not the disease but the man or woman who needs to be treated', then it follows that we should gauge a doctor's worth in part by how well he deals with patients who really annoy him.

Earlier, when I was pissed off with Gimpface for failing to take my septic spot seriously – indeed, for failing to have any idea about what it might be – I sought solace on the internet. I self-diagnosed, as my ancestors would have done, and for a day or so afterwards I granted myself the sick role.

I realise that this was wrong of me. And yet, and yet...

INFORMED CONSUMERS OF HEALTHCARE

Internet health websites and forums exert a pornographic hold on hypochondriacs. Their home pages stress what a fantastic service is being provided, how much our research efforts are empowering us, emboldening us in readiness for our confrontation with The Medical Establishment.

'Drug Infonet provides drug and disease information for your healthcare needs. Visit our FAQ page to find answers to common health questions. Look on the Manufacturer Info page to link to pharmaceutical company pages. Click to Health Info and Health News for the latest in healthcare developments. Drug Infonet brings this free resource to you so that you become a more informed consumer of healthcare.'

The first ever medical encyclopedia was *Firdaws al-hikma* (*Paradise of Wisdom*) by 'Ali ibn Rabban al-Tabari (838-870), one of the founding fathers of Arab-Islamic medicine. It's a seven-volume compendium based on Arabic and Persian translations of Hippocrates and Galen as well as Persian and Indian writers. The most significant volume is Volume Four, which divides into 12 sections, one for each group of ailments: diseases of the head and brain; diseases of the intestines, etc. This would have been the volume hypochondriacs in ninth-century Baghdad lugged around, grumbling 'I wish this had a better index'.

Nowadays, of course, the internet is many people's primary source for health information. A 2003 study by US market research company Harris Interactive found that 109 million adults – 78 per cent of the population of the US – had used the internet for this purpose in the previous year. It's no surprise that doctors resent the internet, and are suspicious of our ability to use it responsibly. It facilitates access to knowledge which, as little as ten years ago, was more or less their exclusive province.

Perhaps this accounts for the snarkiness that pundit-doctors with regular columns in newspapers increasingly show. Readers of the *Times* will be familiar with pseudonymous Essex GP 'Doctor Copperfield', whose yeah-yeah tone suggests that the business of treating ill people is *unbelieeeeeevably*

Level of risk related to exposure to a patient with Lassa fever:

HIGH RISK

o Exposure from a percutaneous injury (eg a cut with a sharp object) to blood, tissue, or other bodily fluids.

o Exposure from direct, unprotected contact with potentially infectious material (eg touching vomitus with an ungloved hand).

o Mucosal exposure (eg of eyes, nose or mouth) to splashes or droplets of potentially infectious blood and bodily fluids.

LOW RISK

o Sharing a room or sitting in a vehicle within six feet (ie, coughing distance) of a potentially infectious patient.

o Providing routine medical care while using personal protective equipment (PPE) appropriately.

o Routine cleaning and laundry of contaminated linens and surfaces.

o Transporting a potentially infectious patient.

o Handling clinical specimens while using PPE appropriately.

Source: National Center for Infectious Diseases, US

tedious. For example: 'Typical, you wait for ages and then three turn up at once. I've spent weeks shepherding hypochondriacs in and out of my consulting room and then, boom boom boom: a bloke with a headache turned out to have had a cerebral haemorrhage; a bow-legged toddler actually had rickets; and a woman presenting with anxiety symptoms now has a newly diagnosed overactive thyroid.' (March 26, 2005)

Correctly judging our relationship with our doctors to be essentially sadomasochistic, commissioning editors are expert at finding columnists who prey on our worst fears. A few years ago, Michael Foxton wrote a series of pseudonymous – these things are always pseudonymous – columns for the *Guardian* laying bare the gruesome details of his traineeship in a London teaching hospital. (They were collected and published in book form as *Bedside Stories* in 2003.) They alerted readers to much that they would probably have preferred not to know. When, for example, a family 'refuse to let the team do the decent thing and put their ageing matriarch "not for resus"', doctors respond, when that matriarch 'crashes', by enacting a 'Hollywood call'. This is when 'the entire cardiac arrest team sprint to the ward, gasping and shouting, bounce up and down on her chest enthusiastically (although delicately enough not to break her ribs) and bark out instructions to each other, giving the stage performance of their lives, before sadly pronouncing to the audience that they did all they could'.

Earlier, I quoted from Raymond Tallis's book *Hippocratic Oaths* a passage in which he expresses serious doubts about the helpfulness of the internet as a health information resource, concluding that 'an "e-hypochondriac" is no more sophisticated than one nourished on glossy magazines'.

Tallis, professor of Geriatric Medicine at the University of Manchester, is a remarkable and respected man who was, in 2004, named one of Britain's 100 most significant intellectuals by *Prospect* magazine. *Hippocratic Oaths* is an impassioned defence not only of scientific medicine, but of the whole idea of medical progress in an era where the NHS is in disarray, surgeons spend more time doing paperwork than operating, and a succession of media controversies (MMR, the retention of children's organs at Alder Hey) has eroded public trust in and respect for the profession to the point where applications for places at medical school have dropped to 1.55 per place from a peak of 3.5. It's a very good book, and only a fool would disagree with the bulk of its conclusions – that, for instance, the prevailing culture of zero tolerance of error will lead to doctors practising 'defensive' medicine out of a fear of litigation; and that people who complain about the 'medicalisation' of society fail to appreciate the way 'old age, death, pain and handicap are thrust on doctors to keep families and society from facing them'.

And yet Tallis is unable to check his irritation with The

Patient – a baffled, bleary figure for whom touchy-feely qualities like 'communication skills' matter much more than doctorly competence.

Tallis reminds us that the people of Hyde initially refused to accept that Harold Shipman was guilty of murder. He'd seemed like the perfect GP – kindly but haggard, worn down by the effort of his daily rounds.

Obviously, no patient wants a docile functionary for a doctor like the one George Bernard Shaw conjures in his preface to *A Doctor's Dilemma* (1911), who, because he 'has to live by pleasing his patients in competition with everybody who has walked the hospitals, scraped through the examinations, and bought a glass plate, soon finds himself prescribing water to teetotallers and brandy or champagne jelly to drunkards… never once daring to say "I don't know", or "I don't agree".'

At the same time, it would be nice to have one who didn't think his patients were incapable of understanding what was wrong with them.

On February 24, 2002, Liz Kendall wrote a piece for the *Observer* titled 'How I fell foul of the NHS'. Kendall had been told that she would need to have her gallbladder taken out, but felt she hadn't been given sufficient information about what the organ did, or if its removal carried risks: 'What does a gallbladder do?' she asked. 'Why does it go wrong? How does the body cope without it?' Her (male) consultant had, she considered, been sexist and dismissive: 'He said it was unusual to find gallstones in someone so young – I was in my mid-twenties – since sufferers are normally "the four Fs: fair, fat, fertile and forty. You're certainly not three of those but hopefully you're still fertile!" I was mortified.'

Tallis quotes her article at length in his book, even remarking in one of the last chapters how rich a resource it's been for him. Kendall's seeming ingratitude to the man who saved her life riles him. The diagnosis was 100 per cent accurate, and her subsequent surgery entirely successful: what, he wonders, is her problem?

You can sort of see his point. There's certainly a whiff of manufactured outrage in Kendall's response to the consultant's insensitive but harmless joke. But what of her complaint that she should have been given more information? Tallis is having none of it: 'The tutorial on the function of the gallbladder and the pathophysiology of gallstones alone would have been quite a major undertaking in the absence of any prior knowledge of biology,' he declares.

This is quite spectacularly patronising. How did the consultant know that Kendall lacked any prior knowledge of biology? And even if she did, it should have been well within his capabilities to explain in layman's terms what the gallbladder is and does. (The word 'pathophysiology' has clearly been slipped in here to annoy.)

Five minutes on the internet is all it takes to find answers to Kendall's questions:

What does a gallbladder do?

The gallbladder is a small organ located just beneath the liver, though connected to both the liver and the small intestine. It stores and concentrates bile. When food arrives in the stomach, a substance called cholecystokinin is released into the blood. This causes the gallbladder to contract, pushing bile into the intestine. This bile is needed to help pancreatic enzymes called lipases digest fat in food and absorb fat-soluble vitamins. It also helps to rid the body of waste products like cholesterol.

Why does it go wrong?

Usually it goes wrong because gallstones form in it. These are solid stones formed from cholesterol, bile salts and calcium. They can vary in size from a few millimetres to a few centimetres. They form when bile contains too much cholesterol. This excess cholesterol creates crystals, and the gallstones are made from these.

How does the body cope without it?

Perfectly well, most of the time.

In terms of the operative risks involved, if the consultant hadn't felt like spelling them out himself, he could always have steered Kendall in the direction of US surgeon Atul Gawande's *Complications: A Surgeon's Notes on an Imperfect Science* (2002) – a wincing litany of front-line screw-ups, most of them Gawande's own, from his days as a trainee. There is a chapter called 'When Doctors Make Mistakes' whose grim centrepiece is a fist-in-mouth – or should that be throat? – account of an emergency tracheotomy. Somehow, because it's Gawande performing it, we know it will be okay. But then he tells us he's only done one before, and that was on a goat…

Later on in this chapter his removal of a dodgy gallbladder prompts the following meditation: 'The stalk of the gallbladder is a branch off the liver's only conduit for sending bile to the intestines… And if you accidentally injure this main bile duct, the bile backs up and starts to destroy the liver. Between 10 and 20 per cent of the patients to whom this happens will die.'

Which is worth knowing.

Perhaps this is glib. Tallis, for one, would say that I am not a typical patient. I am young(ish), university-educated, and I know how to use the internet. I am 'information-literate', broadly able to tell good information from bad. And besides, surfing health sites is an ABC1 thing. As a 2002 report, 'Use of the Internet by Women with Breast Cancer', explains, 'increased income and educational level [are] significant predictors of internet use'.

At the same time, a different research study on the way patients access health information ('The Role of the Internet in Patient-Practitioner Relationships: Findings from a Qualitative Research Study', *Journal of Medical Internet Research*, Vol 6) found that those who used the internet were 'often too overwhelmed by the information available... to make an informed decision about their own care'. It concluded: 'Hype around internet use by patients appears to exceed the reality.'

The problem with this study is the nature of the patients involved. There were 47 in the group – 32 women and 15 men. All the men were being treated for erectile dysfunction; all the women with hormone replacement therapy. As you'd expect, many of them were elderly: the average ages of the men and women were 66 and 55 respectively. Most of them had never used the internet. (Only 29 patients out of 47 had access to it.)

More interesting by far is what the 'healthcare professionals' (their precise status isn't given) interviewed in the report had to say. Some loved the internet and felt it had enhanced patients' understanding of their conditions. Others worried about the dangers of self-diagnosis and 'odd websites'. One person remarked, revealingly, that he often found himself 'having to substantiate some really difficult scenarios where somebody has come armed with this information… You just don't know where to go [and you] haven't got the arguments against their specific topic which they find particularly interesting… You are at a loss: it puts you on your back foot and *makes you feel quite stupid* [my italics].'

The report dares to ask: 'How much, then, were practitioners' concerns about the negative power of the internet a reflection of their own insecurities in its use, and in their own medical competence?' Noting that there were very few instances where patients having acquired information online led to them controlling the outcomes of their consultations, it concludes: 'Clearly, some practitioners were defensive about their own internet competencies. As a result, they asserted their medical authority all the more, thereby dismissing the positive potential of the internet, particularly if the information from it came via a patient.'

PROUST THE JUNKIE

Novelist Marcel Proust suffered badly from asthma and hayfever, and feared social situations that might aggravate his condition. When he was best man at his brother Robert's wedding in 1903, Marcel wore three overcoats, and padded his chest and collar with layers of cotton wool. During the service he had to stand in the aisle because he couldn't fit in the pews.

Both Robert and their father, Adrien, were doctors. Adrien was Professor of the Faculty of Medicine at Paris. His area of expertise was public health, and his most significant achievement the development of the concept of cordon sanitaire to limit the spread of epidemics.

Marcel was closest to his mother. Actually, 'closest' doesn't do justice to the intensity of the relationship. He liked to feel that their lives were perfectly in sync. 'To feel that our sleeping and waking hours are portioned out over one and the same expanse of time will be my delight,' he wrote to her in December 1903. He took care to keep her up to date with assessments of his mental and physical state.

Around 8 per cent of the population of Switzerland suffer from asthma, compared to only 2 per cent 25-30 years ago. According to the UCB Institute of Allergy in Belgium, incidence of asthma in Western Europe as a whole has doubled in the last ten years.

October 22, 1896: 'I think that my feeling so unwell, of which I spoke to you this morning on the telephone, comes partly from my stomach, I mean from the accumulation of the iodine I've been taking, and perhaps from eating inattentively. I'm going to be careful about it...'

August 15, 1902: '[Dr] Vaquez recommended me not to let myself be carried away by morphine (he's no need to be afraid!) or alcohol, which he considers just as detrimental in all its forms. He says he wonders why invalids aren't content with their illnesses, but insist on creating new ones by making themselves unhappy for people who aren't worth the trouble.'

Undated: 'As a precautionary measure you might get some heroin on the offchance, although I'm absolutely determined not to take any. But one can't tell what might happen with these [asthma] attacks, that are so unlike what I've been used to... I feel better at the moment. I hope this rain will put me in better condition. Please get the heroin in any case, just for safety's sake.'

Marcel was hugely incapacitated by his illnesses, but they didn't stop him from challenging to a duel a writer who hinted in a review of the collection of essays, poems and short stories *Les Plaisirs et les jours* that he had enjoyed homosexual relations with the writer Lucien Daudet. The duel was fought on February 7, 1896; both parties fired into the air.

In 1909, after leaving the sanatorium into which he'd checked himself to recover from the trauma of his mother's death in 1905, Marcel started work on what would become *À la recherche du temps perdu* in his apartment on Boulevard Haussmann. He lined his bedroom with cork to reduce noise and dust, and worked through the night, every night, eschewing the comforts of society. The first part, 'Du côté de chez Swann', was published in 1913.

Forced to move from Boulevard Haussmann in 1919, Marcel sold the cork lining to a wine-merchant. By the time he died in 1922, he was taking adrenaline to wake himself up, iodides and stramonium to relieve his asthma, then heroin, Dial, Veronal and Trial to get to sleep.

He died of bronchopneumonia on November 18, 1922. His last word was 'Mother'.

FEIGNED ERUPTIONS

Doctors hate being fooled. This is partly why GPs dislike hypochondriacs so – the suspicion of attention-seeking and game-playing never far away. The delight doctors feel when they unmask a faker is matched only by their impatience with their duped peers.

Francis J Shepherd, a surgeon at Montreal General Hospital in the late 19th century, remembers a famous incident where a man 'simulated locomotor ataxia [syphilis of the spinal cord characterised by degeneration of sensory neurons, stabbing pains in the trunk and legs, unsteady gait, incontinence and impotence] so perfectly that the great Charcot and many other prominent Parisian physicians were deceived'. The man was shunted from hospital to hospital until finally he ended up in

Notre Dame de Lourdes, where he was 'miraculously cured' and 'kept as an example of what Our Lady of Lourdes could do, to the mortification of many members of the medical profession'.

Shepherd, who specialised in skin disorders, had his own share of malingering fakers, as his paper 'Some Cases of Feigned Eruptions' (*Journal of Cutaneous and Genito-Urinary Diseases*, December 1897) makes clear.

'The fact that skin diseases are often feigned is well recognised,' says Shepherd, 'and in some cases the deception is so clever that the fraud may for a long time go undiscovered, especially if the patient falls into the hands of medical men who have no sense of humour, for such are easily imposed upon.' Lupus, for instance, is relatively easy to fake by irritating the skin with tartar-emetic ointment; faux-gangrene by using a rubber bottle filled with hot water.

Amelia B was a 30-year-old servant who had strange circular patches on the backs of her hands and forearms. Some were dry and hard, others shiny and yellowish. 'I at once said that the eruption had been produced artificially,' insists Shepherd, 'but the patient indignantly denied it.' She was admitted to hospital, bandaged and watched to make sure she didn't try any funny business. After one week, the bandages were removed and 'no fresh spots were seen'.

Shepherd's theory? That 'the lesion was evidently produced

by the bottom or cover of some metal box, or other similar article, heated to a high temperature. The object of the trick I could never discover, unless it was to get off her work.'

Another of Shepherd's patients was 28-year-old Laura R who presented 'an eruption on the chest'. Shepherd liked her a lot, taking the opportunity to note her 'considerable intelligence', even if she was 'a nervous woman who had most of the hysterical stigmata'. It transpired that the woman was applying croton oil to her chest 'for some lung trouble'; the suggestion is that she was deliberately irritating the skin on her breasts so that she could present them for medical inspection.

'She seemed to take quite an interest in showing the eruption to the class of students,' Shepherd notes, 'and was not at all abashed in having her breasts uncovered.'

A QUESTION OF RESPECT

Maybe it's just a manner thing. Maybe I shouldn't project, be so defensive, be so suspicious of my doctor's motives. Maybe I should be a nicer person.

I am talking to my friend Paul. Paul is a 41-year-old solicitor from Salford I met on the internet – on a health anxiety forum. I've been impressed by the way he's managed not to alienate doctors with his hypochondria. I wonder how he does it.

'Well,' he says, 'for starters I don't call my doctor Gimpface.'

Paul says he's always maintained respect for doctors. 'I've never wanted to be one of those oh-no-not-you-again patients – the kind doctors talk about among themselves, rolling their eyes. Actually, that's one of the types of reassurance I ask my GP for – reassurance that I'm not annoying him.'

'Does he give it to you?'

'Most of the time.'

Paul admits his affection for his GP may be linked to the man's willingness to refer him when became concerned about a 'change in bowel habits'. Understandably, he thought he had bowel cancer. 'I had to have what I can only call an "invasive procedure", but they were able to give me the all-clear immediately. I felt... euphoria. It was like all my ecstasy hits rolled into one, not that I've had that many. It felt like being reborn, though without the religious connotations. The explanation was irritable bowel syndrome – stress-related irritable bowel syndrome. In other words, I'd been doing this to myself.'

I'm thrilled for Paul. This is great news. I tell him about my brain scan – about how the consultant said I had a '100 per cent normal brain' – and he laughs.

Paul thinks my problem with doctors may be a case of 'classic Freudian transference'. 'Transference' is the idea that distortions in the relationship between a patient and an analyst – or in my case a patient and a GP – will affect the outcome of the treatment. 'People usually talk about transference in terms of someone falling in love with their analyst,' he says. 'But obviously that's not what's happened here.'

'No.'

'It sounds like things with Gimpface have got pretty bad. Maybe they've gone beyond transference.'

'You think?'

'It's possible.'

'Where's that, then – "beyond transference"?'

'Countertransference.'

'Meaning?'

Paul smiles. 'That Gimpface hates you too.'

IN THE PUB

That night, I dream I'm in a pub with Gimpface. It's his local, a pseudo-rustic affair on the outskirts of Croydon. His lordly, jovial manner goes down well here. As we enter he's greeted by the landlord like a long-lost brother. Regulars nod and smile and raise their glasses. A boy playing on a fruit machine turns to his mother at a nearby table and murmurs, 'It's the doctor.' 'He saved your life,' she says, her eyes tracking our progress across the lounge with something close to awe.

Gimpface has bought me a drink – a pint of London Pride. (He favours ice-cold Stella. 'You know where you are with Stella,' he says.) The atmosphere is convivial, the hostility that characterised our past dealings with each other a distant memory.

'This is nice,' I say.

'Yeah,' he says. 'Thought I'd bring you here. Just so you'd, you know... understand me a bit better. So you'd realise that, actually, I'm on your side.'

'You are?'

'Of course. It's a difficult time for you lot – all you worriers. A difficult time in the history of the West. Did you know that in 2000 a survey of psychiatric morbidity carried out by the Office for National Statistics found that one in six adults between the ages of 16 and 74 living in private households had a neurotic disorder – depression, anxiety or a phobia of some sort?'

I shake my head.

'Most of them must know rationally that we're the luckiest and healthiest we've ever been. They must realise that, actually, we should be happy and grateful and turning our thoughts towards the millions of people in the world who don't have clean drinking water or basic drugs. But no.'

I don't know what to say to this. I feel awful (as in guilty, not sick).

'Most people don't go to doctors any more anyway,' he goes on. 'They stay at home and dose themselves with over-the-counter remedies. The US home diagnostic test industry was worth $780 million in 1993, and it's been growing since at a rate of 20 per cent a year, so you can imagine what the figure is now.' He takes a manly gulp of his lager before continuing. 'You came to see me about your prostate, didn't you? You wanted a prostate specific antigen test. I didn't give you one. You got all pissy about it. But tell me, have you any idea how much overtesting goes on? Overtesting which leads, more often than not, to completely unnecessary procedures which represent a far greater risk to the patient's life than the condition they think they're treating. How's your glass?'

'Empty, thanks.'

'Your round.'

I wait at the bar. As he serves me, the barman says *sotto voce*, 'He's a good man, you know.'

'I know,' I say.

'The thing you have to realise,' says Gimpface as I hand him his pint, 'is that there is no conspiracy. All these diseases that people like you bang on about, saying they're evidence of doctors getting it wrong, "200 years ago you thought arthritis was a symptom of hysteria", etc, etc – I'm talking about fibromyalgia, Gulf War Syndrome, environmental hypersensitivity syndrome, ME. Now I'm not saying the people who think they've got these illnesses are lying or malingering or whatever. But the fact is, as far as most of them are concerned, doctors can't find anything wrong. So what are we supposed to conclude? What's our job supposed to be in a situation like that?'

'I don't know,' I say.

'Again, the media fans the flames. I know it's stating the obvious to say how much our culture values youth and beauty and health – glistening, toned bodies. But sadly it bears repetition.' He looks at me, and for a second his subtly aerated hair isn't quite so annoying. 'I'm sorry I didn't spot that your, er, spot was a vascular lesion. I should have done. But the point is, it wasn't cancer. I could see that it wasn't cancer. If it had been cancerous, I would have noticed. Do you see what I mean?'

QUITE INTENSE CRYING

I drift out of sleep and into consciousness, dimly aware of a brittle electronic squawking. I open my eyes and see the lights on the monitor spiking into the red. The alarm clock says 4.06am.

Beside me, Cathy is also awake. She must have woken at the same time. She says, 'That's quite intense crying for her.'

'Her' is our daughter, Scarlett. Ninth months old, she has her mother's blue eyes and blonde hair, and her father's nose and frown. Entirely her own, however, is her eerie serenity. Put her down at night and, more often than not, she'll stretch and smile as if to say 'Ah yes, my cot, good', then sing herself to sleep.

Crying like this means something is wrong. We decide to go in immediately rather than allow her the customary five minutes to resettle herself.

On the two or three occasions when this has happened before – when she's started crying for no obvious reason: maybe a bad dream or teething pain? – we knew everything was okay when the tears abated as soon as we entered and a broad smile greeted us: 'Oh, hi, it's you. Something wrong?'

This time, though, the crying doesn't stop. We flick on the light and the reason becomes clear. There is vomit everywhere – all over Scarlett's hands and face, all over her cot. I am reminded of the episode of *Blake's 7* where the spaceship Liberator is destroyed by a sinister fungal slime.

We are no strangers to Scarlett's vomit. As a small baby she had reflux and would frequently throw up three feeds in a row. It didn't seem to bother her, but for her breastfeeding mother it was tantamount to rejection. I remember returning from work, every day for about two months, to the smell of Dettol and the sound of crying. The doctors just shrugged.

The health visitor who eventually prescribed Gaviscon told Cathy: 'I don't know if this is for her or for you.' Had I been there, I like to think I would have set her straight on that one.

So we understand vomit. We are no longer scared of it – not when it's milky-white, uncurdled, spilling warmly from Scarlett's mouth as if we've simply tilted her too far forward. But this vomit is different. It's semi-digested minestrone soup, foul-smelling and so acidic that it's caused the skin around her mouth to blister.

Carefully, we extract Scarlett from her soiled sleeping bag and pyjamas. We change her nappy (a poo: light-brown, runny). Thinking she must be dehydrated, we offer her water from a bottle which she gulps thirstily.

The conclusion seems inescapable, and inescapably mundane: Scarlett has a tummy bug. But I won't allow myself to believe this. 'Maybe we should take her to A&E,' I say.

Diseases you can tell from observing your poo:

Thin stools – cancer of the rectum or sigmoid colon
White stools – pancreatic cancer
Black stools – stomach cancer, duodenal ulcers, inflammatory bowel disease
Very large stools – Chagas's disease

Cathy looks at me. 'You're kidding.'

'It wouldn't hurt to get her checked out.'

'She's got a bug. There's a nasty one going round. Loads of kids at her playgroup have had it.'

I can't quash the thought. I have to let it out. 'What if it's not a bug? What if it's... stomach cancer?'

'Don't say that.'

'Why not?'

'Because it's hysterical and stupid. It's fine to be a hypochondriac yourself, but don't start projecting on to her.' Her voice softens as she holds Scarlett close, stroking the back of her head. 'She just needs a hug and to go back to sleep. She'll feel better tomorrow.'

Later, when Scarlett has gone back to sleep as quickly as she left it, Cathy says: 'We've got to get used to this. This is going to be a common feature of our lives from now on.'

'I know,' I say. 'It's hard, though, isn't it? To keep everything in perspective. And not to panic.'

AND IN THE END

I don't expect death to be worry-free. Why should it? Nothing about life suggests that death will be any less tedious or complicated or disappointing.

Like most forms of obsessive behaviour, hypochondria is

about asserting control. If I pay close enough attention to my body, I will prevent it being ravaged by illness. If I catch illness early enough, there may be time to cure it. But death doesn't care about control. It doesn't care about prophylactic measures. It will take me when it wants me – in a car, walking in the Lake District, sleeping in a tent at Glastonbury. (Ha! Like I'm *ever* going to sleep in a tent at Glastonbury, the very mention of which mud-saturated germfest transforms me into Bree van der Kamp.) I like to think that my nearest and dearest will see to it that nothing undignified befalls my corpse. But maybe they won't. Maybe they'll decide that, having been fairly useless in life, I might as well have a practical function in death. Let's consider the options:

Dissection by students of gross anatomy
Pros: Tangible benefit to society; saves on funeral costs; the embalming fluid they pump into your veins expands the erectile tissues so it looks like you're really well-endowed.

Cons: You're bound to be mistreated – given a stupid name, left on a bus, etc.

Crime scene experimentation
Pros: Tangible benefit to society; saves on funeral costs; I always liked *CSI*.

Cons: So I'm lying there in a field or in a forest, and a sniffer dog finds me, and because I've been there a while decomposition is quite advanced, to the point where the process known as 'bloat' is under way. Bloat is underway because the bacteria in my now-inactive gut is running riot and feeding on me rather than steak or chicken stew or any other protein that might have been hanging around, waiting to be broken down into amino acids. Bloat is caused by a build-up of trapped gas. It has caused my torso to distend grotesquely so that I am the size of a cow. Not only that, the lower half of my body is almost entirely covered by a writhing, burrowing mass of rice grain-sized maggots. Look: I know this is going to happen anyway. But I don't want a load of people wearing masks and PVC jumpsuits gawping at me while it does. I'd feel really self-conscious.

Ballistics practice
Most of the time, when bullet manufacturers are testing, say, the frangibility (ie, ability to break apart on impact) of bullets, they fire them into the human tissue simulant 'ballistic gelatine'. But occasionally real cadavers are used to test the efficacy of body armour.

Pro: Better than being a crash test dummy.

Con: Better than being a crash test dummy.

Organ donation

This is problematic for hypochondriacs. We believe our organs to be clapped out and not worth transplanting. So what's the point of signing donor cards? It hardly seems ethical – to tease some dying, dialysing teenager with the promise of my manky old kidneys. 'Here you go. One careful user! Don't worry about the lumps, they're only stones.'

I worry about my body's fate. But I worry about my soul, too. I left Catholicism behind a long time ago, but a concept like Hell stays with you. And even though I have committed no worse crime than occasionally overpricing books on Amazon Marketplace, I must confront the possibility that I will end up there. You never know what you might have done to piss God off.

I remember asking Father Douglas about Hell. What was it like? Did a thermostat keep the temperature just so? Was a fiery furnace really the best God could do? What about freezing in carbonite like in *The Empire Strikes Back*?

'Hell is different for everybody,' he said.

'Really?'

'For some people, it might be a room filled with flies or rats. For others it might be a fairground ride where they want to get off but can't.'

He turned his rheumy eyes towards me. 'What bothers you most in life?'

I thought, but didn't say: 'The idea of a prolapsed rectum.' I did say: 'Illnesses I might get.'

'Well then,' said Father Douglas. 'Maybe your Hell will involve being horribly ill. Or maybe it will involve thinking you're horribly ill. That can be almost as bad.' He chuckled – heesheesheesh. 'The important thing is to trust in the Lord. Only He decides when we're ill and when we're not, just as only He decides when it's time for us to die.'

'What if I deliberately ran in front of a car?'

'That would be the will of God working through you.'

***

But you see, this doesn't work for me. I can't leave my physical wellbeing in the hands of an imaginary God. Voltaire found it impossible to believe in the God who had allowed the Lisbon earthquake of 1755 to happen. I find it impossible to believe in a God who would allow me to get skin cancer, which may just be solipsism on my part but hey.

What, then, is the upshot?

It is that I must – we must – be vigilant. We must stand before the mirror and inspect ourselves, every last fold and crease, for lumps and gristly bits and misshapen spots, and we must do this regularly, and we must take our findings to our GPs because you never know.

You never know. But there's a slim chance they might.

USEFUL NUMBERS

Mental Health Foundation
020 7802 0300
www.mentalhealth.org.uk

British Association for Behavioural and Cognitive Psychotherapies (BABCP)
01254 875277
www.babcp.org.uk

British Association for Counselling and Psychotherapy (BACP)
0870 443 5252
www.bacp.co.uk

Samaritans
08457 909090
www.samaritans.org.uk

NHS Direct Online
www.nhsdirect.nhs.uk

BIBLIOGRAPHY

It felt inefficient to list here books already cited in the text, though I have given a second mention to those I thought especially important. These are, for the most part, books I used for broader research. Of the few books that exist about hypochondria, the best are probably Susan Baur's *Hypochondria: Woeful Imaginings* (University of California Press, 1988) and Carla Cantor and Brian Fallon's *Phantom Illness: Shattering the Myth of Hypochondria* (Houghton Mifflin, 1996). Baur's book, especially, steered me in the direction of Darwin, Boswell and much besides. Anyone wishing to pursue the subject further (not to say more seriously) should start there. *Hypochondriasis: Modern Perspectives on an Ancient Malady* (Oxford University Press, 2001), a collection of essays edited by Vladan Starcevic and Don R Lipsitt, was also helpful. Much of the material relating to Darwin and Proust is sourced from George Pickering's excellent *Creative Malady* (Allen & Unwin, 1974).

As far as more general books about medicine are concerned, no home should be without Roy Porter's *The Greatest Benefit to Mankind: A Medical History of Humanity From Antiquity to the Present* (Fontana, 1997) or – another Porter production – *The Cambridge Illustrated History of Medicine* (Cambridge University Press, 1996).

Kingsley Amis, *Memoirs* (Hutchinson, 1991)

Ralph Colp, *To Be An Invalid* (University of Chicago Press, 1977)

Russell Davies (ed.), *The Kenneth Williams Diaries* (HarperCollins, 1993)

George Frederick Drinka, *The Birth of Neurosis: Myth, Malady and the Victorians* (Simon & Schuster, 1984)

Judith Flanders, *The Victorian House* (HarperCollins, 2004)

Michael Foxton, *Bedside Stories: Confessions of a Junior Doctor* (Guardian/Atlantic, 2003)

Atul Gawande, *Complications: A Surgeon's Notes on an Imperfect Science* (Profile, 2002)

Richard Gordon, *The Alarming History of Medicine* (Sinclair-Stevenson, 1993) (for the anecdote about digitalis) Helen King, *Greek and Roman Medicine* (Bristol Classical Press, 2001)

A Lloyd Moote and Dorothy C Moote, *The Great Plague: The Story of London's Most Deadly Year* (John Hopkins University Press, 2003)

Andrew Motion, *Philip Larkin: A Writer's Life* (Faber, 1993)

Adam Phillips, *Terrors and Experts* (Faber, 1995)

Roy Porter (ed), *The Faber Book of Madness* (Faber, 1991)

Jennifer Radden (ed), *The Nature of Melancholy: From Aristotle to Kristeva* (Oxford University Press, 2000)

Gwen Raverat, *Period Piece* (Faber, 1952)

Mary Roach, *Stiff: The Curious Lives of Human Cadavers* (Penguin, 2004)

F Clifford Rose and M Gawel, *Migraine: The Facts* (Oxford University Press, 1979)

Elaine Showalter, *The Female Malady: Women, Madness and English Culture 1830-1980* (Virago, 1985)

Andrew and Penny Stanway, *Pears Encyclopedia of Child Health* (Pelham, 1979)

Raymond Tallis, *Hippocratic Oaths* (Atlantic, 2004)

Claire Tomalin, *Samuel Pepys: The Unequalled Self* (Viking, 2002)

The Modern Family Doctor (TC&EC Jack, 1914)

THANK YOU

Cathy Newman; Antony Topping; Sathnam Sanghera; Nicholas Royle; Alice Fisher; Alex Heminsley; Jonathan Derbyshire; Martina Hladka; Alex O'Connell; Patricia Earl and Brian O'Connell; Peter Earl; Julia and David Newman; Rebecca Nicolson and Aurea Carpenter at Short Books; Laura Lee Davies, Chris Hemblade, Gordon Thomson, Jessica Cargill Thompson and all at *Time Out*. Thank you to Faber & Faber for permission to quote from Philip Larkin's 'Aubade'.

NOTE

In the memoir sections, some names and other distinguishing details have been changed to protect privacy and spare embarrassment.

Norfolk's Win

by river, road and rail

Luke Bonwick

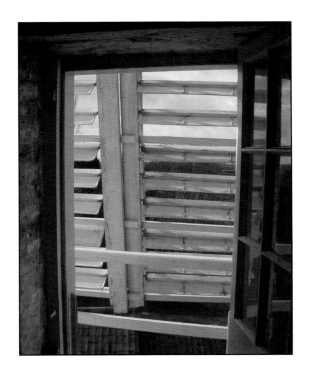

Bonwick Publishing
www.bonwick.co.uk
2008

Norfolk's Windmills by river, road and rail

Published by Bonwick Publishing - www.bonwick.co.uk

©Luke Bonwick 2008

ISBN 978-0-9556314-0-5

Printed by Riverside Press Ltd., Ipswich, Suffolk - www.riversidepress.co.uk

A note on mapping

The nine original maps used in the book are not drawn to scale and are designed to be used as tools to help pinpoint the mills, rather than as accurate navigational aids. Most of the mills described are marked on the recent Ordnance Survey maps - of particular use are the 1:25,000 Explorer editions.

Front cover photo: Turf Fen Mill, How Hill, by Mike Page

Acknowledgements

All photographs and drawings used in the book are protected by copyright. Unless listed below, these are from the author's collection. My sincere thanks go to the following people and organisations for supplying photographs and drawings and for permission to include them in the book (numbers refer to pages):

Peter Allard	12 (upper)
Kathy Beale	Title page, 7 (both), 9 (both), 25
The Broads Authority	13
Adrian Colman	39 (left)
Mildred Cookson	6 (top), 17 (top), 20, 41, 44 (left), 67 (upper)
Eastern Daily Press	14, 17 (lower), 45 (lower)
Ecotricity	68, 69 (lower), 70
Barre Funnell	8
Roger Hough	19 (top right), 30
Mills Archive Trust	12 (lower), 40 (upper), back cover
Jonathan Neville	43
Norfolk County Council / The Norfolk Windmills Trust	18, 21 (lower), 40 (lower), 53, 55 (both), 56 (both), 62, 64 (left)
Mike Page	Front cover, 52 (upper), 63
Vincent Pargeter	21 (upper)
Dave Rogers	61
Richard Seago	16 (right)
Robert Seago	52 (lower)
Andrew Stacey	69 (upper), 71 (upper)
Anne Wagstaff	57
James Waterfield	49 (lower)
Jim Woodward-Nutt	67 (lower)

Particular thanks are due to Kathy Beale, Madeline Carroll, Mildred and Ron Cookson, Barre Funnell, Gareth Hughes, Sheila Hutchinson, Sylvia Lawn, Ken and Helen Major, Bob Paterson, Bryan Read and Dave Pearce for their contributions and advice regarding production of the book. A number of people have looked over the text in detail and suggested improvements and additions. I am especially grateful to Vincent Pargeter, Richard Seago and Alison Yardy for their detailed comments and for sharing their close knowledge of Norfolk mills. Thanks are also due to my wife and family for their unstinting encouragement and help.

Contents

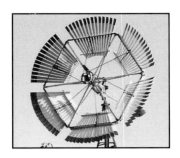

PART 1: BACKGROUND INFORMATION

1.1   Introduction

The corn and drainage windmills of the Norfolk countryside are unique in the UK.

As picturesque reminders of a bygone way of life, many examples have now been restored to their former glory. Most of the mills welcome visitors and open their doors during the summer months, allowing their interiors to be explored. All of them stand close to public roads or waterways and their exteriors can be clearly seen, whatever the season or the weather.

This book is designed as a guide to visiting each of the mills and understanding them in the context of their naturally beautiful surroundings. It takes a detailed look at 15 corn windmills, 18 drainage windmills and a handful of 'unusual' mill sites, as well as the modern successors to the traditional windmill. It also describes some of the personalities involved in the operation, repair and restoration of these mills over the last 150 years.

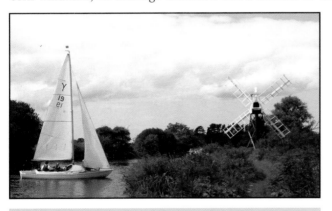

BOARDMAN'S WINDMILL *on the River Ant at How Hill*

Most of the mills can be reached by road, although the mills of north Norfolk and Broadland are perhaps best appreciated by bicycle, so why not leave the car behind? In Broadland you can hire a boat at many of the waterside locations and approach the drainage mills by river. Several drainage mills can be clearly seen from the train, including the recently-restored pair at Seven Mile House on the River Yare and the famous Berney Arms windmill which is several miles from anywhere!

The county's mills have been split into several small groups so you can visit them easily within an afternoon. Each section of the expanded gazetteer includes an area map which indicates where the mills are located in relation to roads, towns and places of significance. Details of how to find the mills are shown on each map. Separate tours describe the corn and drainage windmills in the West Norfolk area; along the coast of North Norfolk; in the area surrounding the Broads and in South Norfolk, close to the Suffolk border.

1.2 Corn milling by wind power

Background

Once, almost every other parish in Norfolk had its own windmill. The late Harry Apling estimated that, at their peak in the mid-19th century, some 420 windmills were at work in the county. Certain parishes, such as Burnham Overy near the northern coast, have more than one windmill, and others, such as Billingford near the Suffolk border, can claim a succession of mills on the same site.

More than forty references to 13th-century windmills in Norfolk have been discovered. Most of these examples were located in the southern half of the county; the earliest of these was a windmill at Norwich which existed in 1235. The earliest portion of a windmill survives as part of an unusual house at Briningham. Known as the Belle Vue Tower, it was built in the 18th century on the brick base of an octagonal smock mill which had been erected in 1721.

The two main types of windmill to be found in Norfolk, the post mill and the tower mill, could be applied to perform a range of industrial functions. A windmill's rotating sails convert the power of the wind into kinetic energy to operate machinery and perform useful work. In Norfolk, windmills were mainly used either to grind corn into flour or to drain water from the low-lying marshland.

In the case of a corn windmill, the mill's four sails are connected, via a system of gears inside the mill, to one or more pairs of *millstones*. Wheat or other grain is fed into the millstones and is ground into meal, or flour, as it passes between them. Only the upper of the two millstones rotates; the lower one remains stationary and a wooden casing around the stones catches the flour as it emerges. The 'wholemeal' flour can either be used as it is, or sieved by a *dressing machine* to produce white flour and other grades. Most windmills operated two or three pairs of millstones, although Old Buckenham Mill is exceptional in having five pairs on one floor.

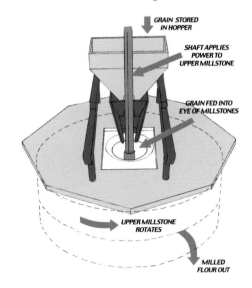

GRAIN STORED IN HOPPER

SHAFT APPLIES POWER TO UPPER MILLSTONE

GRAIN FED INTO EYE OF MILLSTONES

UPPER MILLSTONE ROTATES

MILLED FLOUR OUT

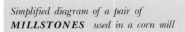

Simplified diagram of a pair of **MILLSTONES** *used in a corn mill*

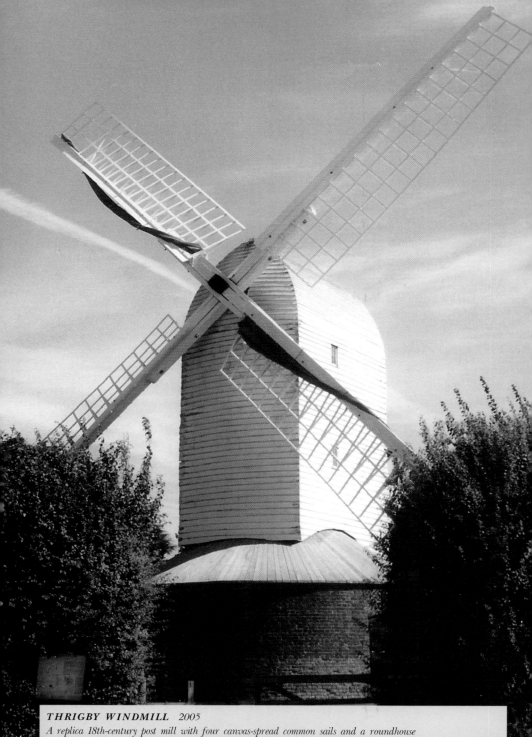

THRIGBY WINDMILL *2005*
A replica 18th-century post mill with four canvas-spread common sails and a roundhouse

The post mill

A typical Norfolk *post mill*, such as Thrigby Mill, is composed of two parts: a timber-framed, weatherboarded body - known locally as the *buck* (1) - supported by a substantial timber *trestle* (2). In the photograph of Thrigby Mill, the trestle cannot be seen as it is enclosed by a circular brick *roundhouse* (3). This protects the trestle from exposure to the elements and provides additional storage space.

The post mill derives its name from the large upright *main post* of oak (4) - the principal timber of the trestle - on which the mill's buck is balanced. The design of the post mill allows the entire buck to rotate through 360° around the post, enabling the mill's *sails* (5) to face the wind from whichever direction it is blowing.

The mill's four sails are attached at the front, or head, of the buck. A large *ladder* (6) attached to the rear, or tail, provides access to the milling machinery inside. The *tailpole* (7), a large timber lever, projects through the tail ladder. In order to turn the sails to face the wind, the miller needed to put his back to the tailpole and push the entire mill round.

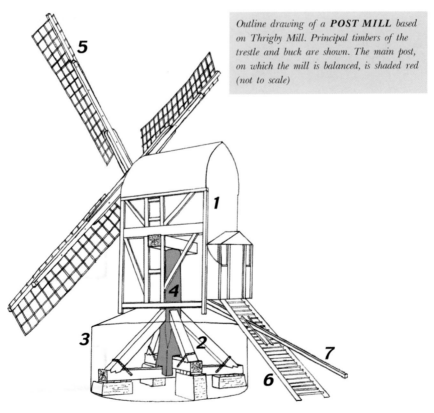

Outline drawing of a **POST MILL** based on Thrigby Mill. Principal timbers of the trestle and buck are shown. The main post, on which the mill is balanced, is shaded red (not to scale)

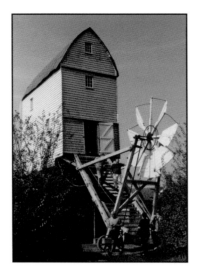

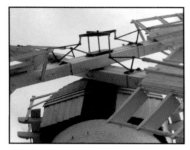

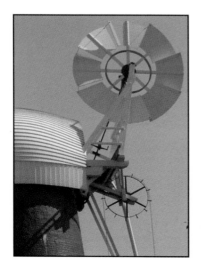

Sails and fantails

Thrigby Mill is fitted with four *common sails* which had to be spread with canvas in order to catch the wind. The miller would do this by hand, stopping each sail at its lowest position and, if necessary, climbing the sails to secure the canvas with ropes. Common sails are time-consuming, difficult and sometimes dangerous to use, particularly in squally weather. With too much canvas on the sails, the mill could run too fast and become out of control, with the risk of severe damage.

Many post mills, such as Garboldisham Mill, were modernised to improve their efficiency as new technologies became available. In place of the tailpole, Garboldisham Mill (top left) has a *fantail* which automatically steers the buck towards the wind whenever it changes direction. The fantail, locally known as the 'fly', comprises a set of small blades set at right angles to the main sails that will rotate in either direction as soon as the wind veers. The fantail was patented in 1745 and, by the early-19th century, was becoming increasingly more popular in Norfolk.

Another important invention was a new design of sail, patented in 1807 by William Cubitt, the son of a Norfolk miller. In the style of a Venetian blind, Cubitt's *patent sails* contained a series of adjustable shutters or *vanes* which could be closed to catch the wind or opened to allow it to pass between them. Its advantage over the common sail was that, using a system of centrally-controlled rods, the vanes in all four sails could be adjusted simultaneously, without the need to stop the mill.

(top) **Fantail** *attached to the ladder of a post mill*
(middle) **Patent sails**, *with adjustable vanes operated by cranks and rods*
(bottom) **Fantail** *attached to the cap of a tower mill. The control gear for a set of* **patent sails** *can be seen underneath the platform below the fantail*

The tower mill

During the 19th century, many of Norfolk's post mills were replaced by a more advanced design of windmill, the *tower mill*. With this type of mill, the driving gears, millstones and machinery are contained in a stationary tower, built of brickwork in the form of a truncated cone. On top of the tower rests the timber-framed *cap*, to which the sails are attached, and this alone can rotate to allow the sails to face the wind.

Tower mills could vary considerably in height and stature. Norfolk's earliest tower mills, built during the 18th century, tended to be no more than three storeys in height in order that the sails and winding gear could be reached from ground level. Just like a primitive post mill, the first tower mills used a braced *tailpole* - extending downwards from the cap - to turn the sails into wind (see p12). The fantail and the patent sail are ideally suited for use with a tower mill as they do not require adjustment from ground level. This advantage gave millwrights the freedom to build much taller, more powerful and more elaborate windmills than had previously been conceivable (see p21).

The drawing of Denver Mill shows the internal layout of a typical large tower mill. The mill's four *patent sails* swing well clear of ground level and are adjusted by chains which hang down from the rear of the cap. A narrow walkway, or *reefing stage*, encircles the second floor of the mill and gives access to these chains for adjustment. The brake, used to start and stop the sails of the mill, is also controlled by a chain from the reefing stage. A similar walkway, known as the *gallery*, surrounds the mill's ogee cap, making maintenance at this height much easier.

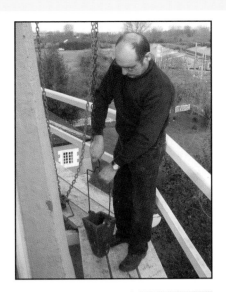

*Miller Chris Garner hangs a weight on the chain which operates the vanes in the sails at **DENVER MILL***

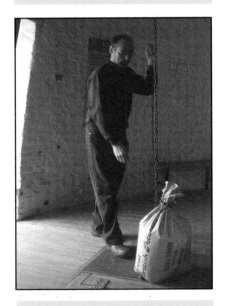

Chris hangs a sack of grain on the hoist chain at the bottom of the mill. It is lifted to the top by wind power

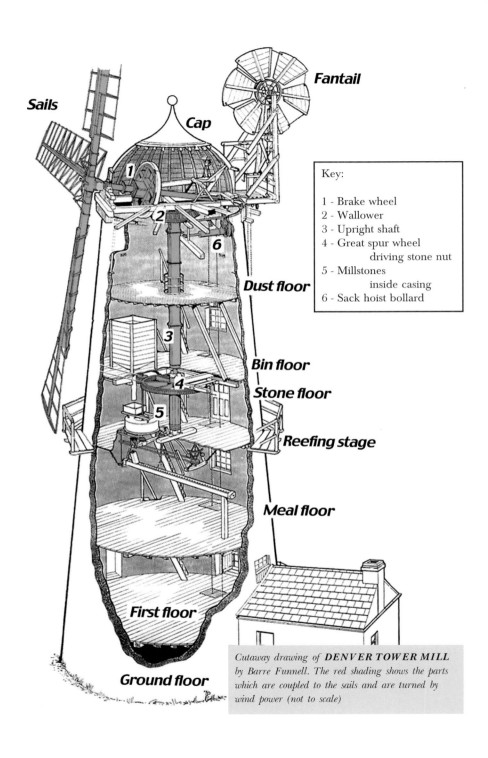

Sails

Fantail

Cap

Key:

1 - Brake wheel
2 - Wallower
3 - Upright shaft
4 - Great spur wheel
    driving stone nut
5 - Millstones
    inside casing
6 - Sack hoist bollard

Dust floor

Bin floor

Stone floor

Reefing stage

Meal floor

First floor

Ground floor

*Cutaway drawing of **DENVER TOWER MILL** by Barre Funnell. The red shading shows the parts which are coupled to the sails and are turned by wind power (not to scale)*

The *fantail*, which steers the ogee cap around to face the wind, is mounted on a timber framework at the rear of the cap. The cap rotates on a circular track, the *curb*, on top of the tower brickwork. A system of reduction gears link the fantail to a toothed ring attached to the curb. The fantail is very sensitive to changes in wind direction and can be rotated by the pressure of a finger. A few revolutions of the fantail will move the cap round only slightly; over 1,000 revolutions are needed to turn it through 360°.

Three pairs of *millstones* are situated on the third floor, and the great spur wheel which drives them is positioned directly above. This is known as an 'overdrift' arrangement and may be compared with the layout of Sutton Mill, where the millstones are 'underdrift'. A long *upright shaft* passes through the centre of the mill, linking the great spur wheel to the primary gears inside the cap, three floors above. At the top of the upright shaft is a bevelled gear wheel, the *wallower*, which engages the larger *brake wheel* mounted on the inclined cast-iron windshaft. The relative sizes of the gear wheels mean that the millstones will rotate at up to 120 rpm - more than ten times faster than the sails.

Every mill, particularly a tall one, needed a *sack hoist* to relieve the miller of the arduous task of carrying grain up several flights of stairs to the level of the millstones. The sack hoist consists of a stout, cylindrical *bollard*, rotated by wind power, around which a chain is wound. A sack, secured to the end of the chain on the ground floor, can be drawn upwards through trapdoors set above one another in each floor. Sacks of grain are hoisted to the *bin floor* above the level of the millstones, and milled flour is collected from a spout on the *meal floor* below them.

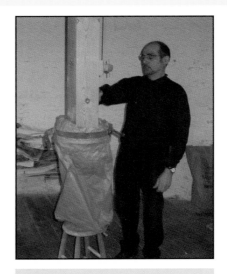

Milled flour descends through a spout from the millstones into a waiting sack. Chris checks the fineness of the flour being produced between finger and thumb

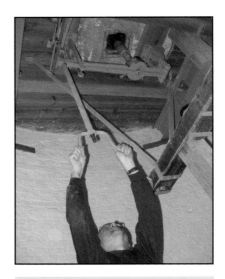

By adjusting the tentering screw, Chris can alter the working gap between the two millstones to make the milled flour coarser or finer

1.3 Land drainage by wind power

Background

Norfolk's low-lying marshlands make ideal grazing and farming land, provided they can be drained of excess water and kept relatively dry. A Dutch engineer, Cornelius Vermuyden, took responsibility for the drainage of England's Fens in the mid-17th century. Over the following century, the first references to windmills being used for drainage in Norfolk begin to appear. During the second half of the 18th century, wind-powered drainage mills gradually became established in Broadland. Faden's map, published in 1797, shows 47 of them and this number had increased to an estimated maximum of between 100 and 140 a century later. Today, the remains of more than 70 drainage windmills can be found in the Norfolk and Suffolk Broads, although several of these sites are only accessible to the most intrepid of explorers. By contrast, almost all the mills in the fenlands of Cambridgeshire and Lincolnshire have disappeared without trace.

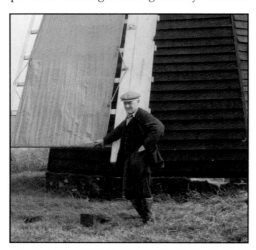

Charlie Howlett, the last marshman at **HERRINGFLEET DRAINAGE MILL**, *seen setting the common sails in the 1950s*

The working life of a marshman

An area of drained marsh was known as a *level* and contained a network of dykes which channelled water towards the mill. A drainage mill could be named after the level it drained, the landowner it belonged to or the marshman who operated it. The size of a level varied considerably; some were very small, while others could cover 1000 acres (404.7 hectares).

The mills would be kept working whenever the marshes needed draining and there was sufficient wind to turn the sails. To the marshmen, this often meant long, arduous night shifts. An old-fashioned mill, like High's Mill at Halvergate (see p12), would need constant monitoring to ensure it did not run too fast or too slowly and that it always faced into the wind. A more up-to-date example, such as Stracey Arms Mill (see p53), would adjust itself automatically as it worked and could largely be left to its own devices, allowing the marshman to concentrate on his other duties. These included managing the grazing livestock, cleaning out the dykes and principal waterways every year, and maintaining the desired water level.

Devices for lifting water

The drainage windmills that can be seen today used three different devices to raise water from the marshland into the rivers. The *scoop wheel* (see p67) is the simplest and most commonly found device. It comprises a series of wooden paddles set in the form of a large wheel. The scoop wheel rotates inside a brick culvert and its upper part is enclosed by a boarded timber *hoodway*. Water enters at one end of the culvert, emerging at a higher level at the other. The scoop wheel can raise water three-eighths of its diameter - most usually between 3 and 5 feet (0.91 - 1.52 m).

Mr Appold patented the *turbine pump* in the mid-19th century. This was half as efficient again as the scoop wheel, although less reliable in gusty wind conditions. The Appold turbine consists of an impeller, with a number of curved blades, fitting inside a circular casing. Water is drawn into the impeller and is flung out by centrifugal force, rising inside the casing to exit at a higher level than it entered at. England's, millwrights of Ludham, favoured the turbine and the majority of mills fitted with them had been built, or worked on, by England's.

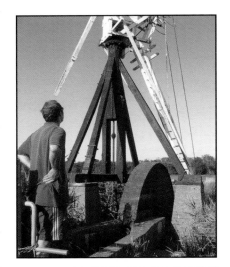

The *plunger pump*, fitted to some mills, comprised a piston inside a cylinder set in the ground. The piston was operated by a crank rod and lifted water trapped in the cylinder to a higher level.

Development of the drainage mill

In order to adapt the post mill for marshland drainage, the problem of transferring power from the top of the mill to the bottom had to be overcome. This was achieved by drilling a hole down the centre of the main post to accommodate a rod or shaft.

*Base of a **hollow post mill**. The slim shaft, seen emerging from the base of the main post, drives a scoop wheel inside the semicircular hoodway*

Early Broadland *hollow post mills* had a crank rod attached directly to the windshaft, which operated a simple plunger pump set in the ground underneath the mill. Later mills, such as Clayrack Mill at How Hill (above), had a gear wheel on the windshaft which rotated a vertical shaft that passed through the main post to drive a scoop wheel.

During the 18th century, when the first tower-type drainage mills began to appear in Broadland, limited technology was available. Old photographs of some of the surviving early mills, such as High's Mill at Halvergate, show their simple features. The common sails on High's Mill had to be manually spread with sheets of canvas; its cap was winded by a braced tailpole and chain winch; its internal machinery was largely of wood and of very primitive construction. In operation, these early mills were time-consuming and often hard work for the marshman in charge. By comparison, a thoroughly modern late-19th century mill such as Stracey Arms displays many of the improvements fitted to make the marshman's job easier. Its patent sails would be largely self-regulating once

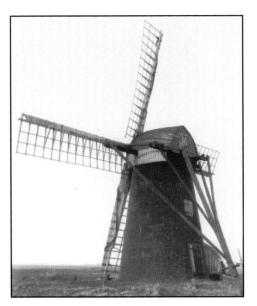

HIGH'S DRAINAGE MILL, HALVERGATE, *1944. A primitive tower mill. Its four common sails and braced tailpole, with a hand winch to wind the mill, can be seen*

they had been set initially, and its fantail compensated automatically for any variations in wind direction during the working day. Its internal machinery, being largely of cast iron, reduced the frequency of breakdowns due to the failure of wooden gear cogs.

The relatively high cost of building a substantial brick tower mill may have led some millwrights to develop more cost-effective alternatives which made use of the same technology. *Skeleton mills*, such as Boardman's Mill at How Hill, are miniature tower mills in essence, the tapering brickwork being substituted for open timber frameworks which were quicker, and much cheaper, to erect.

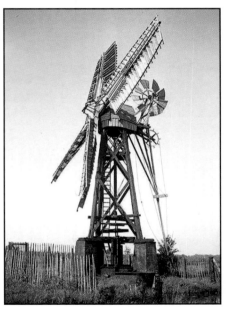

BOARDMAN'S SKELETON MILL *at How Hill in working order, 1934. The shaft which passes down the centre of the mill to drive a turbine pump can be seen. The mill was originally fitted with a scoop wheel*

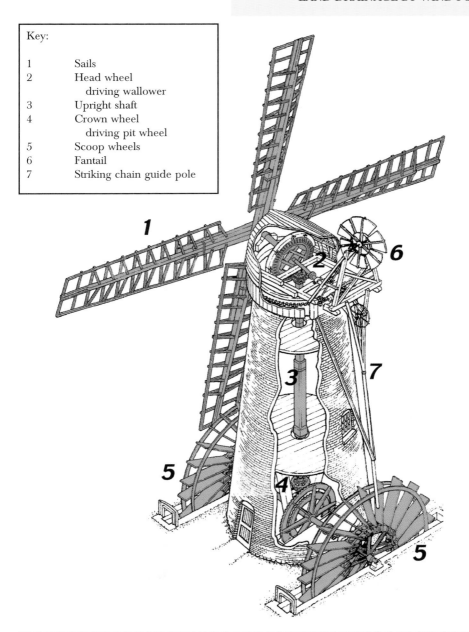

Key:

1	Sails
2	Head wheel driving wallower
3	Upright shaft
4	Crown wheel driving pit wheel
5	Scoop wheels
6	Fantail
7	Striking chain guide pole

*Cutaway drawing by Alan Batley showing a conjectural **brick-built drainage mill** driving twin scoop wheels. The red shading shows the parts which are coupled to the sails and are turned by wind power. The sail vanes and their operating gear have been omitted from the drawing (not to scale)*

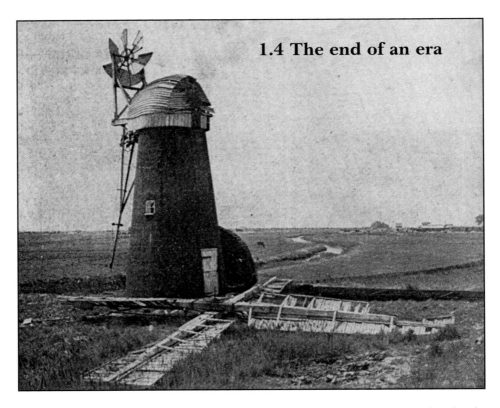

1.4 The end of an era

The rapid development of fossil fuels and more efficient modes of transport during the 19th and early-20th centuries brought the use of corn milling by wind power to an end. The number of working corn windmills in the county had declined from an estimated peak of 425 in the mid-19th century to 100 by 1912, 11 by 1937 and only one in 1956.

The drainage mills of Broadland experienced a similar decline, as power sources which had worked alongside wind power gradually superseded it. In 1946, all seven mills on the Halvergate Fleet were made redundant by the installation of an electric pump at the head of the channel. Drainage of the northern Broads using wind power was brought to a disastrous end on 1st January, 1953, when the sails of Ashtree Farm Mill (above) were destroyed in a violent storm. This little mill has been a well-known landmark since it was built in 1912; it stands close by the River Bure and is clearly visible to motorists travelling between Acle and Great Yarmouth. Although the mill stood derelict for nearly fifty years, the damage has now been rectified as a result of the recent 'Land of the Windmills' project. Organised by Norfolk Windmills Trust and funded by substantial grants from the Heritage Lottery Fund and other organisations, this scheme has enabled three drainage windmills and a steam-engine house in the Broads area to be restored for the benefit of local residents and visitors to the region.

1.5 New beginnings

Pioneering Preservationists

One of the leading lights of the movement to restore Norfolk's windmills was Rex Wailes (1901-1986). An engineer by profession, Rex became the country's recognised authority on windmills soon after visiting his first one in 1923. He campaigned tirelessly for their preservation throughout his life. In 1955, the Norfolk County Planning Department asked Rex to report on the condition of the surviving windmills in the county. A list of 18 mills was arrived at and, following the selection of priorities, the restoration movement swung into action. The survey was undertaken in partnership with Jack Thompson, the head of a firm of millwrights from Alford in Lincolnshire (see p16).

The Norfolk Windmills Trust was established in 1963 with the aim of preserving selected examples of corn and drainage windmills for the benefit of future generations. Funded by a regular grant from the County Council, the Trust has, in the past, been assisted by generous donations from the Broadland boat firms, District and Parish Councils, national and local bodies, private companies and members of the public.

Arthur C. Smith was the first enthusiast to undertake comprehensive surveys of all the surviving remains of corn and drainage windmills in the county, the results of which were published in the 1970s and 80s (see p72). Most remarkably, Arthur covered the hundreds of miles necessary to complete the surveys by bicycle!

Old-time millwrights

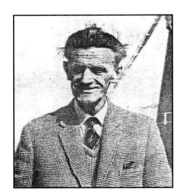

CECIL SMITHDALE
seen at Berney Arms, c1970

The role of the millwright, who built the mills and carried out running repairs to them, was a fulfilling although challenging one. The millwright's job combined the skills of carpenter, engineer, blacksmith, mason and design draughtsman. It required work with bare hands, often in confined spaces and in adverse weather conditions. The achievements of the old-time millwrights, who built windmills up to 11 storeys tall and over 100 feet (30.5 m) in height, are all the more remarkable when one considers that they had no mobile cranes or modern power tools to help them. Hefty cast-iron shafts and gears and huge baulks of timber had to be transported to site, unloaded and hoisted into place using only pulley blocks, ropes, levers - and teamwork.

Famous firms of Norfolk millwrights such as England's of Ludham and Smithdale's of Acle have been outlasted by the mills they built. In 1965-67, when in his sixties, Cecil Smithdale supervised the restoration of Berney Arms tower mill for the Ministry of Works. The family firm carried out millwrighting, engineering, iron and brass founding and implement making; it had been established in Norwich in 1853 by Cecil's grandfather, Thomas.

Contemporary millwrights

Happily, a number of skilled craftsmen have kept the millwrighting trade alive into the 21st century. Although not all of them can be included here, certain individuals deserve special mention.

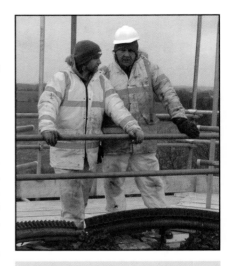

R. Thompson & Son of Alford, Lincolnshire, is the last of the UK's old millwrighting firms still in operation. Founded in 1877, Thompson's was latterly run by its foreman, Jim Davies, who took over in the 1970s following the death of Jack Thompson. Jim's son, Tom Davies, now runs the business. Following the 1955 survey, Thompson's undertook many of the early restorations including the county's first - at Billingford - and are still restoring Norfolk mills today.

Steve Boulton (left) and Tom Davies from **R. THOMPSON & SON** *at work in Essex, 2007*

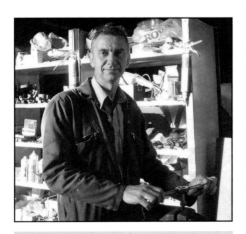

RICHARD SEAGO seen at South Walsham, 2007

Richard Seago, born and bred in the county, has worked on more than 30 corn and drainage windmills. In 1977, at the age of 18, he rescued and began to reconstruct his first windmill, the small drainage windmill at Upton Dyke. Since then he has built several new caps for drainage and corn mills. Richard's own replica post mill at South Walsham, which he started building in 1994, is now nearly complete.

The late John Lawn, another Norfolkman and former RAF engineer, began his professional millwrighting career in the early 1970s. Almost every windmill in the county received John's attention in the

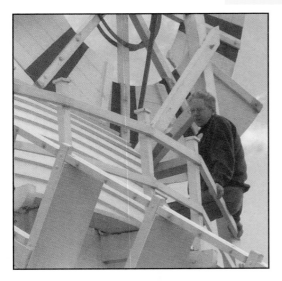

VINCENT PARGETER
at Thurne Mill, 2004

following three decades. Initially working in partnership with Philip Lennard of Essex, and later with the assistance of Adrian Bond of Wymondham, John successfully retrieved several important mills from the brink of dereliction. His most memorable restorations include the spectacular corn mills at Old Buckenham and Wicklewood, and the picturesque Turf Fen drainage mill at How Hill.

As a boy, Vincent Pargeter, a native of Kent, became familiar with the sight of Norfolk's windmills on summer holidays to the Broads with his parents. Forty years on, his unrivalled knowledge of water- and windmills is supported by a wealth

of practical restoration and repair work. Together with his assistant, Bob Self, Vincent has returned the drainage mills at Seven Mile House and Thurne to working order. In his spare time, Vincent has rescued and rebuilt a traditional clinker-built Norfolk wherry.

Of equal importance to Norfolk's mills have been several volunteer millwrights who have taken on the restoration of their own individual mills. The Norfolk landscape owes much to these dedicated teams and individuals - too numerous to mention separately - who have sought to preserve their own mills as part of the rural scene.

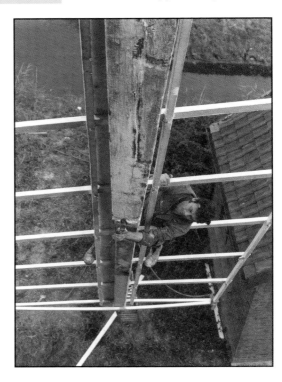

JOHN LAWN
seen at Stracey Arms, 1976

1.6 Technical facts and figures

Variety and contrast

One of the reasons why the study of mills is so interesting is that every mill was built as a one-off and no two are exactly alike. Each of the mill builders, or *millwrights*, had different ideas about the best type of mill to build. Some preferred the traditional post mill, constructed entirely of wood and balanced on a stout central post. Other millwrights favoured the more solid brick tower mill, which could be built taller and so catch more wind. A cheaper, though less durable, alternative to this design was the *smock mill*, in which timber was substituted for brick as the main building material.

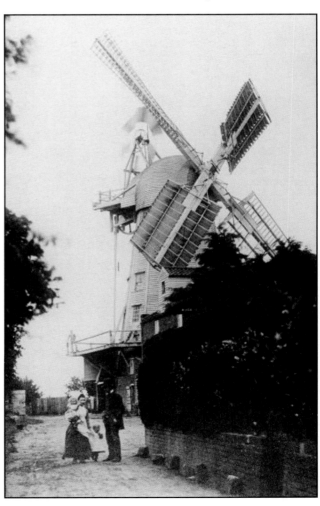

The different 'signatures' of each millwright can be seen by comparing the exterior features of mills from different areas of the county. The great variety of wooden caps on the mills demonstrate these local styles well. In the west of the county, in the area surrounding The Wash, many mills had onion-shaped or *ogee caps*, circular in plan, clad in vertical weatherboarding and surmounted by elegant finials.

COOKE'S WINDMILL, STALHAM 1888
This large timber-framed smock mill was one of the first windmills in the UK to be fitted with William Cubitt's patent sails. It was completely destroyed by fire in 1903.

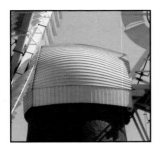 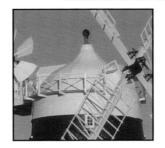 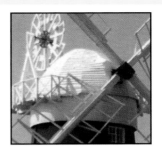

(left to right) Boat-shaped cap, **POLKEY'S MILL, REEDHAM MARSHES**; *ogee-shaped cap,* **SAVORY'S MILL, BURNHAM OVERY**; *dome-shaped cap,* **STOW MILL, PASTON**

Around the north coast, a number of polygonal, almost *dome-shaped caps* are found. The predominant and instantly recognisable form of Norfolk cap is the *boat-shaped cap*. Its elegant and streamlined appearance is very pleasing in profile. It is constructed in a similar way to an upturned boat with paired, curved rafters, horizontal weatherboarding and a petticoat of short, vertical boards around the base. Viewed in elevation, the cap's ridge could be straight and level or curved and falling from front to rear.

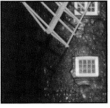 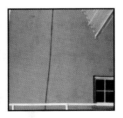
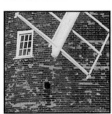 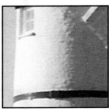

(clockwise from top left) **BURNHAM OVERY MILL; DENVER MILL; THURNE MILL; OLD BUCKENHAM MILL**

Many Norfolk mills had a walkway or *gallery* around the eaves of the cap to allow access for maintenance. Variations in the design of the gallery handrails give each cap a slightly different character. Burnham Overy Mill has a white-painted timber cap gallery with decorative cross-bracing to the handrail; a sharp contrast is provided by Great Bircham Mill (p27) which has a wrought iron gallery and presents a more austere appearance. The elegant curves of the cap are more accentuated on mills such as Polkey's which do not have a cap gallery. Different fantails can also be seen, many with six or eight blades but some - more unusually - with seven or even ten. Millwrights tried different means of excluding the weather from the mills they built. Towers could be covered with cement render and then painted, as at Denver; whitewashed as at Thurne; tarred as at Burnham Overy or simply left with bare brickwork, as at Old Buckenham. White lead paint, containing linseed oil, was the favoured means of protecting woodwork from driving wind and rain.

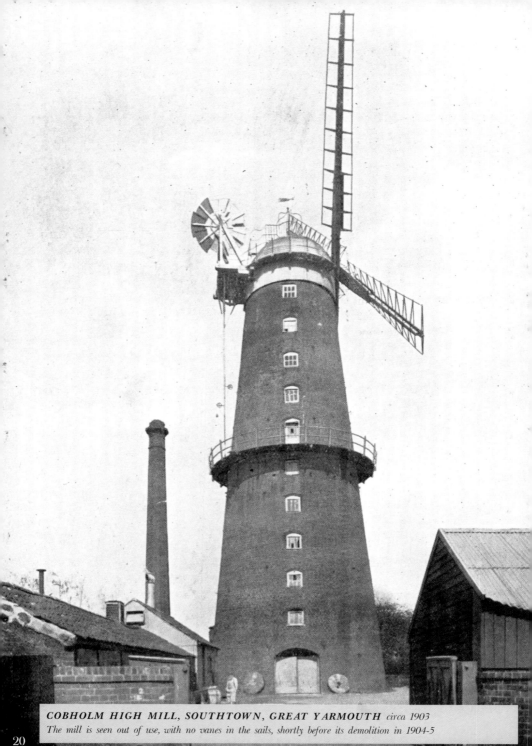

COBHOLM HIGH MILL, SOUTHTOWN, GREAT YARMOUTH *circa 1903*
The mill is seen out of use, with no vanes in the sails, shortly before its demolition in 1904-5

Norfolk's Giants

Norfolk, perhaps more than any other county in England, gained a reputation for its many large and powerful windmills. Though very few of these record-breaking giants can still be seen today, we are fortunate that a number survived into the era of the photographer. Several historians - no doubt impressed by the engineering of these huge structures - have recorded important details of Norfolk's tallest windmills for posterity.

The most famous of all the Norfolk giants was Cobholm High Mill at Southtown, a suburb of Great Yarmouth. During the late-19th century it was owned and run by the successful milling firm of Press Brothers. The enormous mill, built in 1812, was 11 storeys high and stood 112 feet (34.14 metres) tall. Given its great height, the mill was an important 'seamark' for shipping.

High Mill was not the tallest windmill ever built in Norfolk, however. This honour goes to Bixley Mill near Norwich, the lower part of which still survives.

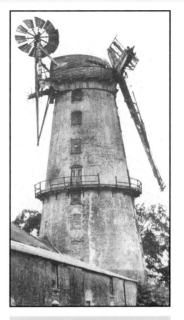

SUTTON WINDMILL
Derelict, in the 1960s, after being struck by lightning

Until 1865, when it was dismantled and the materials sold at auction, Bixley Mill stood an incredible 137 feet (41.76 metres) tall. The mill may have been simply too large to handle - the reason for its demolition was that it failed to make a profit.

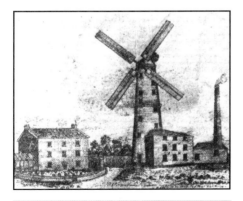

BIXLEY WINDMILL, the tallest ever built in the county, during its heyday in the mid-19th century

At just under 79 feet (24.38 m) to the ridge of the cap, Sutton Mill, near Stalham, is the tallest windmill still standing in East Anglia. Its height is accentuated by the run of windows and door openings in the tower, which are set one above the other. The brick tower, cap and sails were all painted white during the mill's working days and must have presented a splendid sight. Since it ceased work in 1940 following damage from a lightning strike, the mill has been partly restored. It is hoped that the recent work carried out by the Nunn family can be continued in the future, and the mill made to work again.

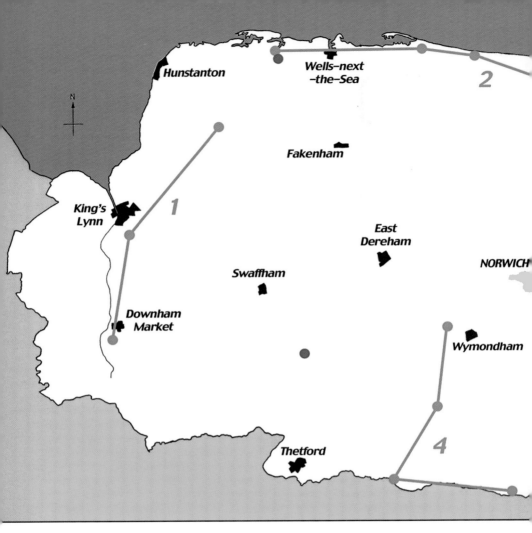

Key:

1 - West Norfolk Corn Mills tour
2 - North Norfolk Corn Mills tour
3 - Broads Area Corn Mills tour
4 - South Norfolk Corn Mills tour

5 - River Ant Drainage Mills tour
6 - River Thurne Drainage Mills tour
7 - River Bure Drainage Mills tour
8 - River Yare Drainage Mills tour
9 - River Waveney Drainage Mills tour

Unusual Mill sites

For the current opening times of the mills, please refer to locally-published literature. Visiting information is also available at **www.bonwick.co.uk**

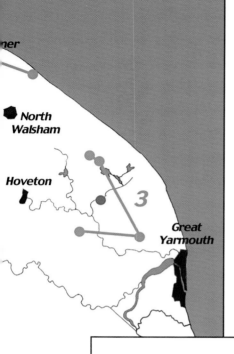

ner

North Walsham

Hoveton

3

Great Yarmouth

PART 2:
TOURING THE COUNTY

Left: Map of the county
showing the locations of the corn mills
and the unusual mill sites

Below: Enlarged map of the Broads area
showing the locations of the drainage mills

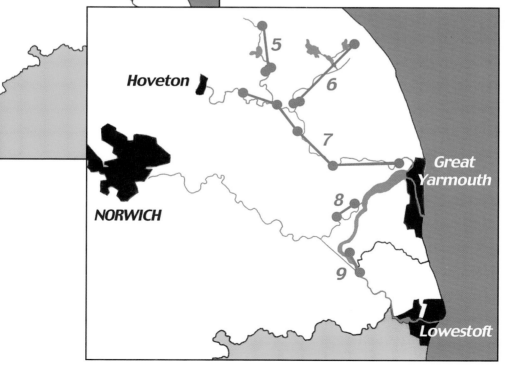

Hoveton

5

6

7

8

9

NORWICH

Great Yarmouth

Lowestoft

Corn Mills of West Norfolk

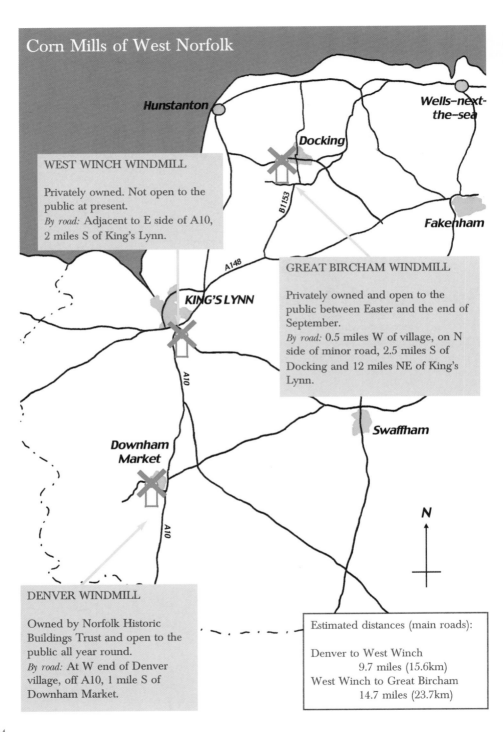

Hunstanton

Wells–next–the–sea

Docking

Fakenham

B1153

WEST WINCH WINDMILL

Privately owned. Not open to the public at present.
By road: Adjacent to E side of A10, 2 miles S of King's Lynn.

A148

KING'S LYNN

GREAT BIRCHAM WINDMILL

Privately owned and open to the public between Easter and the end of September.
By road: 0.5 miles W of village, on N side of minor road, 2.5 miles S of Docking and 12 miles NE of King's Lynn.

A10

Swaffham

Downham Market

N

A10

DENVER WINDMILL

Owned by Norfolk Historic Buildings Trust and open to the public all year round.
By road: At W end of Denver village, off A10, 1 mile S of Downham Market.

Estimated distances (main roads):

Denver to West Winch
9.7 miles (15.6km)
West Winch to Great Bircham
14.7 miles (23.7km)

2.1 Corn Mills of West Norfolk

Denver Mill TF 605012 (see pages 7-9)

*At 59 feet (17.9 m) to the top of its rendered brick tower, Denver **tower mill** is the largest survivor of the tall fenland windmills.*

The mill stands in a traditional rural setting, together with its collection of original outbuildings including a granary, an engine house, the former steam mill and the original miller's house. This substantial tower mill is six storeys in height and had a 106-year working life, being built to replace a post mill in 1835. By 1863 it had been joined by a 12 horse-power steam mill. After ceasing work by wind power in 1941, Denver mill was deliberately preserved in good order by its last miller, Thomas Edwin Harris. Following extensive refurbishment, the mill is now fully operational. Inside the mill, two pairs of overdrift millstones and a flour dresser are powered by the sails and can regularly be seen at work. There are four patent sails, an ogee cap with a gallery and a six-bladed fantail. When the mill was repainted recently, 100 litres of masonry paint were needed for the tower.

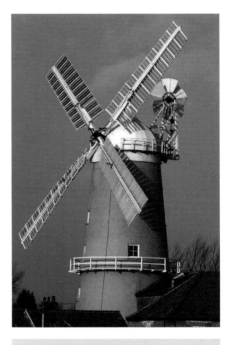

DENVER WINDMILL 2006

West Winch Mill TF 631167

*Joined onto this **tower mill** is the former bakehouse - now a residence - with an unusual cut-out section in its roof. This allowed the sails of the windmill to turn without colliding with the building.*

A well-proportioned tower mill of five storeys, it was built circa 1821 and by 1855 had been fitted up with three pairs of stones and auxiliary machinery driven by patent sails. At this time a horse mill worked in conjunction with the windmill. Over the next ten years the thriving business was enlarged with the addition of a granary, workshop and bakery, and a steam engine drove a fourth pair of stones in the windmill. The use of wind power was abandoned in 1926 but business at the site ceased altogether when, in 1937, 51-year-old miller Ernest Kerrison met a grisly fate when he became entangled in the turning machinery.

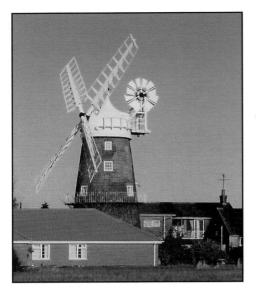

Local builder Walter Price purchased the ivy-covered ruin of the mill in 1973 and it was repaired as a landmark. The first step towards restoration of the mill to working order was made by the present owners, John and Rose Owen, on 10th June 2004, when the cap and sails were lowered to ground level for repair.

Inside the mill, three pairs of millstones were overdriven by a cast-iron great spur wheel. The windshaft and brake wheel are entirely of cast iron. At second-floor level an iron reefing stage gives access to the brake- and striking chains. An interesting feature of the mill is the downpipe and circular gutter around the top of the tower which collect excess water from the cap's petticoat.

WEST WINCH WINDMILL 2002

Great Bircham Mill TF 760326

*Perhaps the most spectacular windmill in Norfolk, Great Bircham **tower mill** has beautiful proportions and a splendid traditional atmosphere inside. It was the first restored windmill in the county to work again by wind power.*

The tower was constructed by George Humphrey in 1846; an early photograph shows the mill's cream-coloured bricks which later received a coat of tar. Between 1883 and 1888 the miller at Bircham was Joseph Wagg, great-grandfather of the mill's restorer.

Roger and Gina Wagg purchased the derelict wreck of the mill in September 1975 and set about restoring it. They were assisted by millwright John Lawn, who dismantled the remaining woodwork and proceeded to build and fit a new ogee cap, six-bladed fantail and four new sails mounted on hollow steel stocks. A new clasp-arm brake wheel was built to engage the iron wallower. Searches at derelict mills in the locality produced second-hand machinery to replace items missing at Bircham. On the second floor, one pair of stones is in working order, overdriven by a large cast-iron spur wheel and stone nut. A forked lever can be used to lower the stone nut down its shaft and out of mesh with the spur wheel. The sails and their operating gear can be reached from a wooden reefing stage surrounding the tower at second-floor level. Adjoining the mill are the original coal-fired bake ovens. Visitors can climb right to the top of the mill and emerge outside on a platform just below the turning fantail.

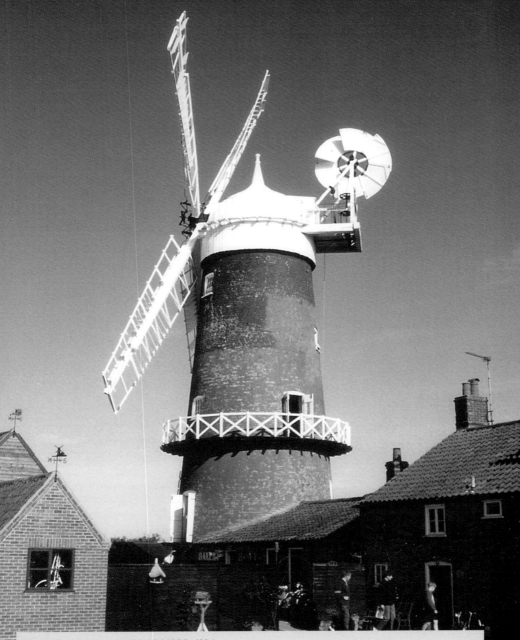

GREAT BIRCHAM WINDMILL *1994*
A mid-19th century tarred brick tower mill with patent sails, ogee-shaped cap and fantail

Corn Mills of North Norfolk

BURNHAM OVERY, SAVORY'S WINDMILL

Owned by the National Trust. Not open to the public.
By road: Adjacent to S side of A149, 0.5 miles W of Burnham Overy and 1 mile N of Burnham Market.

CLEY WINDMILL

Privately owned and open all year round as a guesthouse.
By road: Behind houses in centre of village, on N side of A149.

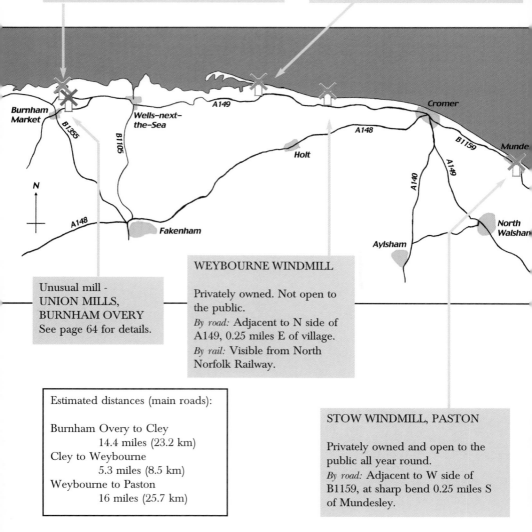

WEYBOURNE WINDMILL

Privately owned. Not open to the public.
By road: Adjacent to N side of A149, 0.25 miles E of village.
By rail: Visible from North Norfolk Railway.

Unusual mill -
UNION MILLS, BURNHAM OVERY
See page 64 for details.

STOW WINDMILL, PASTON

Privately owned and open to the public all year round.
By road: Adjacent to W side of B1159, at sharp bend 0.25 miles S of Mundesley.

Estimated distances (main roads):

Burnham Overy to Cley
    14.4 miles (23.2 km)
Cley to Weybourne
    5.3 miles (8.5 km)
Weybourne to Paston
    16 miles (25.7 km)

2.2 Corn Mills of North Norfolk

Burnham Overy, Savory's Mill TF 837437

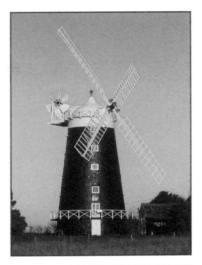

*Burnham Overy is the only Norfolk parish to boast a windmill, a watermill and a combined wind- and watermill. The most prominent of these is the large black **tower mill** which overlooks the marshes near Burnham Overy Staithe.*

Dating from 1816, the mill worked for 98 years and was converted to holiday accommodation early in the 20th century. Today, owned by the National Trust, it can still be rented by holidaymakers although it is not open for general inspection by the public. The mill has a fine ogee cap with a gallery around it, four shutterless patent sails and a six-bladed fantail. The tower is six storeys high and a narrow reefing stage with elegant cross-bracing encircles the mill at first-floor level.

SAVORY'S WINDMILL, BURNHAM OVERY 2006

Cley next the Sea Mill TG 044440

*According to one author, the famous **tower mill** at Cley is "probably the most painted and photographed mill in the country". It appeared on a popular BBC television sequence with a red and yellow hot air balloon, when its sails could be seen turning.*

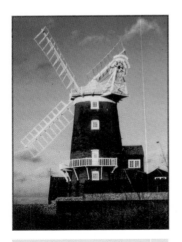

CLEY WINDMILL 1995

Cley was the first windmill on the Norfolk coast to be converted to living accommodation - as early as 1921. In a beautiful setting overlooking the mud flats, Cley mill epitomises the rural corn mill. It was built in 1819 and its three pairs of millstones worked hard in their time for a succession of tenant millers. The retired mill, which ceased work in 1917, is run as a guesthouse and is maintained in excellent condition, but its cap is fixed in one direction and there are no longer millstones inside for the sails to turn. Fortunately, the fine wooden clasp-arm brake wheel survives. The cap is an unusual polygonal dome, surmounted by a ball finial, and the eight-bladed fantail is painted white with a red stripe. There is a timber gallery around the cap and a wooden reefing stage at second- floor level.

Weybourne Mill TG 115431

*Part of an old wooden post mill, which once stood nearby, has been built into the house attached to Weybourne **tower mill**. A lockable "miller's cash box", with a wooden cover 8 inches (20 cm) square, can still be seen cut into this timber.*

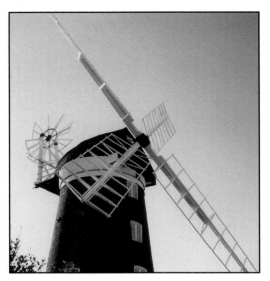

WEYBOURNE WINDMILL 1994

Superbly positioned overlooking the coast road, Weybourne mill can be seen from the nearby steam railway which runs between Sheringham and Holt. The mill is a typical mid-19th century example which became derelict in the 1920s and was stripped of its machinery. Fortunately the cast-iron windshaft, which supported the sails, was spared and now carries four sails once again. A new black boat-shaped cap, which replaces the white-painted original, was built by local craftsmen in 1968. The sails and fantail are 'skeletonised', with no shutters or boards, to protect them from being damaged by the strong winds often experienced in this exposed location. The mill is five storeys high and originally had a reefing stage at second- floor level.

Stow Mill, Paston TG 316357

*Stow Mill is a small brick **tower mill** of four storeys and stands in a prominent position on a hill overlooking the holiday retreat of Mundesley on Sea. An old photograph shows the mill with a white-painted tower, though it is now tarred to protect it from the weather.*

When the mill was built, between 1825 and 1827, it had common sails which swept close to the ground and had to be furled by hand. After grinding corn into meal for over 100 years, the millstones and dressing machinery were stripped out in the early 1930s by new owners who wanted to use the mill as a residential annexe to their house. Restoration

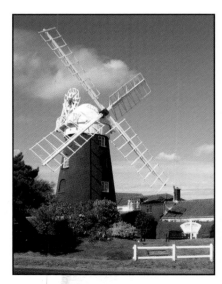

PASTON WINDMILL 2007

of the mill began in 1961 with the aid of a grant from Norfolk County Council. The work was continued in the 1970s and 1980s by enthusiastic owner Mike Newton and his wife Mary, who installed machinery salvaged from other mills to replace missing parts. The mill now has four patent sails without shutters and a 'skeleton' fantail. Of the internal machinery, the brake wheel, wallower and upright shaft are in position. The polygonal dome-shaped cap has a wooden gallery around it although, unlike the cap of Cley Mill, it has no central finial.

STOW WINDMILL, PASTON circa 1890
The mill at work, showing the tower in its original white-painted form

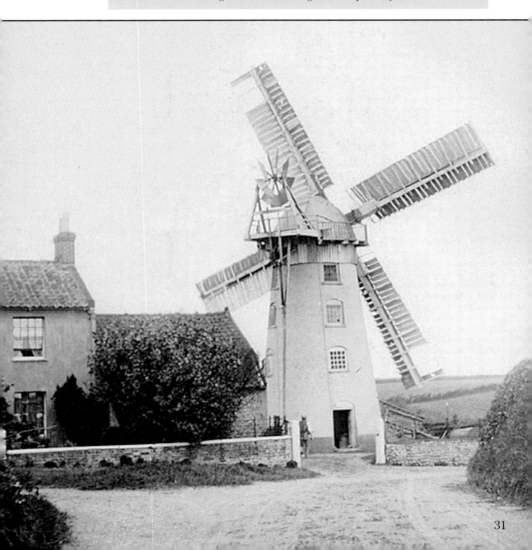

Corn Mills of the Broads Area

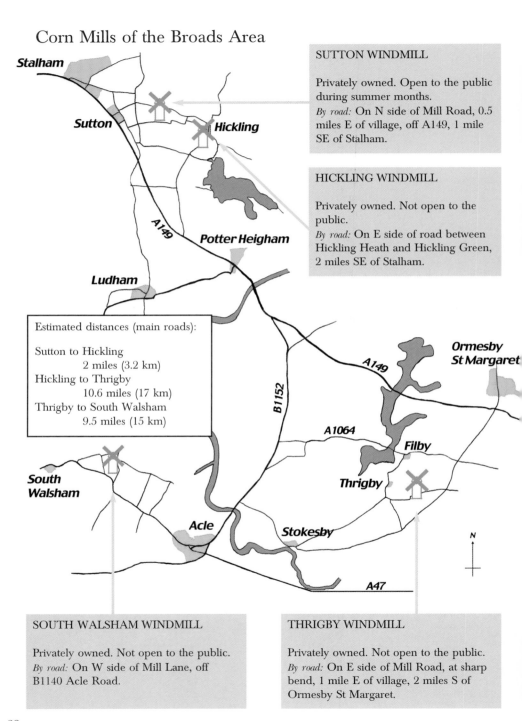

SUTTON WINDMILL

Privately owned. Open to the public during summer months.
By road: On N side of Mill Road, 0.5 miles E of village, off A149, 1 mile SE of Stalham.

HICKLING WINDMILL

Privately owned. Not open to the public.
By road: On E side of road between Hickling Heath and Hickling Green, 2 miles SE of Stalham.

Estimated distances (main roads):

Sutton to Hickling
     2 miles (3.2 km)
Hickling to Thrigby
     10.6 miles (17 km)
Thrigby to South Walsham
     9.5 miles (15 km)

SOUTH WALSHAM WINDMILL

Privately owned. Not open to the public.
By road: On W side of Mill Lane, off B1140 Acle Road.

THRIGBY WINDMILL

Privately owned. Not open to the public.
By road: On E side of Mill Road, at sharp bend, 1 mile E of village, 2 miles S of Ormesby St Margaret.

2.3 Corn Mills of the Broads Area

Sutton Mill TG 395238

*This **tower mill** is Norfolk's tallest surviving windmill. It is nine storeys high and measures almost 80 feet (24.38 m) to the top of its cap. Its four patent sails spanned 73 feet (22.25 m).*

Sutton mill stands on the site of a previous tower mill, itself quite a large structure. Following a disastrous fire in 1861, the present mill was completed the following year and for much of its life was operated by the Worts family. Lightning set the sails of the mill on fire in 1940, ending its working life. When purchased by the Nunn family in 1975, the mill was on the brink of dereliction. Thirty years on, in spite of much positive work, it is again in need of extensive repair.

The red brick tower, rendered and painted white during the mill's working days, is 67 feet 6 inches (20.57 m) high and tapers from 33 feet (10 m) diameter at ground level to 16 feet (4.88 m) at the curb. A narrow reefing stage encircles the tower at fifth-floor level and a gallery surrounds the boat-shaped cap. The fantail, unusually, had ten blades - a characteristic signature of the work of the 19th century millwright Daniel England of Ludham.

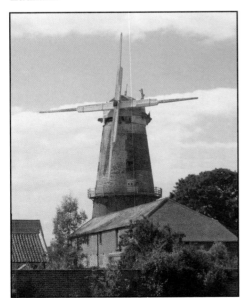

SUTTON WINDMILL 2006
The rustic centrepiece of a fascinating museum of country bygones

On the fifth floor are four pairs of millstones, each 54 inches (1.37 m) in diameter. An additional pair, now removed, were located on the second floor and driven by a long countershaft. The surviving millstones were 'underdrift' - driven from beneath by a cast-iron great spur wheel and four smaller stone nuts, which can be examined on the fourth floor. On the seventh floor, an iron crown wheel on the upright shaft transmitted power to the sack hoist. From the eighth floor, the fine cast-iron brake wheel and wallower can be seen.

In addition to the five pairs of millstones, this powerful windmill could run three flour dressing machines, a maize cutter, an oat roller and a grindstone for sharpening tools.

Hickling Mill TG 408230

*A splendid, early-19th century **tower mill** of eight storeys. The mill's height is exaggerated by the run of windows set one above the other, and the fact that there is no reefing stage encircling the tower.*

The mill was probably built shortly before 1818 and was worked by a succession of tenant millers. One of these, by the name of Israel Royal Garrett, was a farmer and merchant and also owned a bakery, in addition to running the mill. The last miller, Henry Wright, had given up the mill by 1904. Early postcards show the mill already missing its sail vanes and fantail blades.

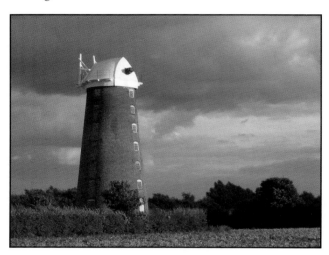

HICKLING WINDMILL 2006
A fine red-brick tower mill, preserved and almost complete

Today, the mill remains in the ownership of the Forbes family, who acquired the property in 1934 and have since maintained it in a fine state of preservation. The cap and fanstage were rebuilt by millwright Richard Seago in 1989-90, but the ten-bladed fantail and four patent sails have not been refitted. The mill contains a fine set of timber gearing. Three pairs of French burr millstones were overdriven on the fourth floor. The great spur wheel has been increased in diameter to speed up the millstones, perhaps when patent sails were first installed. The unusual and well-designed sack hoist, with its integral cone clutch, survives on the dust floor.

Thrigby Mill TG 468120   (Illustration: page 4)

*Norfolk's first 're-born' **post mill**, it was built between 1982 and 1985 by Nick Prior, who painstakingly re-created the mill from its brick roundhouse upwards.*

The post mill at Thrigby appears on Faden's 1797 map, although its precise date of construction is not known. The last miller was Alfred Charles Hood who gave up trading and had the mill dismantled in 1892. For many years, all that remained of the mill was the brick roundhouse containing the worm-eaten trestle timbers. These were copied in new oak and placed on the original brick piers. The wooden body, or buck, of the mill was reconstructed on the ground nearby and then hoisted onto the trestle. Inside, two pairs of millstones and smaller fittings have gradually been added to create an authentic atmosphere. New sails completed the external appearance of the mill in 2004. The sails have been fitted with canvas to allow them to idle in the breeze. In a few years' time corn will again be ground at Thrigby Mill.

South Walsham Mill TG 379129

*This is Norfolk's newest 'old mill' - a replica **post mill** of traditional regional design. It stands near the site of an old post mill which disappeared as long ago as 1870.*

The white-painted buck contains three floors and sits above a circular red brick roundhouse of two storeys. In November 2000, a mobile crane lifted the buck onto the centre post. The mill's builder, professional millwright Richard Seago, has restored many mills in Norfolk. He began building the mill in 1994. Although the timber structure of the mill is entirely new, several iron components from long-destroyed East Anglian mills have been incorporated in the construction.

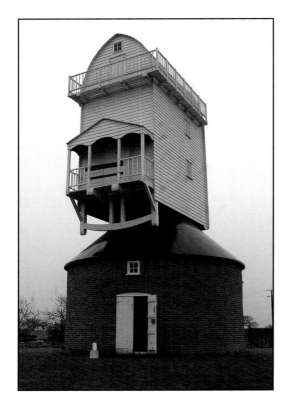

SOUTH WALSHAM WINDMILL
2006
The roundhouse and buck are finished and await the tail ladder and sails

South Walsham windmill has several local characteristics. It will be the only post mill in the county with a fantail mounted on a carriage at the end of its tailpole. This feature, common to several mills in Norfolk, was also popular in Sussex where two examples can be seen today. The last mill in Norfolk with a 'tailpole fantackle` was Tottenhill Mill near Kings Lynn, demolished in 1961. Like Tottenhill, South Walsham mill has a walkway, or gallery, around the eaves of the roof. There is also a decorative porch above the rear door, similar to that at Thrigby Mill.

Corn Mills of South Norfolk

OLD BUCKENHAM WINDMILL

Owned by Norfolk County Council and open to the public during summer months.

By road: S of village green, off B1077, 5 miles SE of Attleborough.

WICKLEWOOD WINDMILL

Owned by Norfolk County Council and open to the public during summer months.

By road: Off B1135, approx 2.5 miles W of Wymondham.

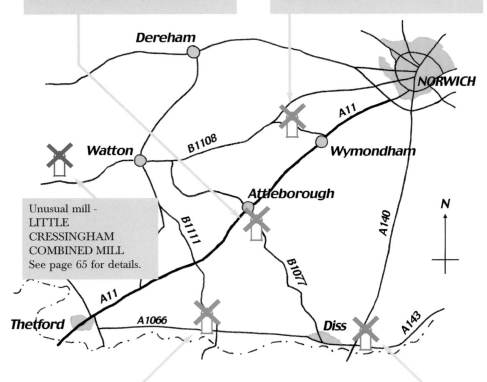

Dereham

NORWICH

Watton

B1108

A11

Wymondham

Attleborough

Unusual mill - LITTLE CRESSINGHAM COMBINED MILL See page 65 for details.

B1111

A140

N

B1077

A11

Thetford

A1066

Diss

A143

GARBOLDISHAM WINDMILL

Privately owned and open to the public by appointment.

By road: On S side of B1111, 1 mile S of village, S of A1066.

BILLINGFORD WINDMILL

Owned by Norfolk County Council and open to the public during summer months.

By road: On common by A143, 1 mile E of junction with A140 at Scole.

Estimated distances (main roads):	Wicklewood to Old Buckenham	8.4 miles (13.5 km)
	Old Buckenham to Garboldisham	8.7 miles (14 km)
	Garboldisham to Billingford	9.5 miles (15.3 km)

2.4 Corn Mills of South Norfolk

Wicklewood Mill TG 076026   (Illustration: back cover)

*By 1977, a roofless ruin was all that remained of Wicklewood **tower mill**. Thanks to the generosity of Margaret Edwards, grand-daughter of the last miller, the mill was given to Norfolk County Council, and the Norfolk Windmills Trust acted quickly to arrest the decay of the structure. Restoration began in 1979.*

This picturesque village mill was built in 1845/46. There are four patent sails, a six-bladed fantail and a boat-shaped cap with a gallery. An unusual feature of the 5-storey mill is the fine wooden roller, suspended below the third floor, which was part of the apparatus used to lift apart the heavy millstones when their working faces needed re-cutting. Two pairs of millstones were driven by wind power and an additional pair were powered by a 12/14 h.p. Shanks paraffin engine. The engine was sold by the last miller after the mill ceased work in 1941, but it has recently been returned to the site.

Old Buckenham Mill TM 062909

*The dimensions of this impressive **tower mill** make it a countrywide record-breaker. It has the largest cap, the most pairs of millstones on one floor and the widest sails of any windmill in the UK.*

The red brick tower has an internal diameter of 26 feet 6 inches (8 m) at the base and 23 feet (7 m) at the top. Above it, the enormous boat-shaped cap is 24 feet (7.32 m) wide. The four patent sails are 10 feet 4 inches (3.15 m) wide and have a diameter of 79 feet (24.1 m). The mill also has the largest known great spur wheel in a windmill - a 12-piece iron casting, 13 feet (3.96 m) in diameter, with 171 teeth.

The sites of six former windmills have been traced in Old Buckenham. The present tower mill was built in 1818 to replace a succession of post mills. When construction began the best available materials were used, but as it progressed upwards these declined in quality as the owner's finances became stretched! A large granary, now house converted, was built next to the mill in 1856; this incorporated a steam mill with four pairs of stones driven by a 12 horse-power engine. In the 19th century the mills were owned by J. & J. Colman, the mustard manufacturers. The last miller, William Goodrum, had an arm amputated in 1921 after being injured by the machinery, but it was the loss of the fantail in 1926 that finally prevented him from working the mill. The remains of the sails and cap were removed in 1976 by local millwright John Lawn, but it was not until 1992 that he could start work on a full restoration, which was completed in 1996. A plaque at the door of the mill commemorates John, who died in 1999.

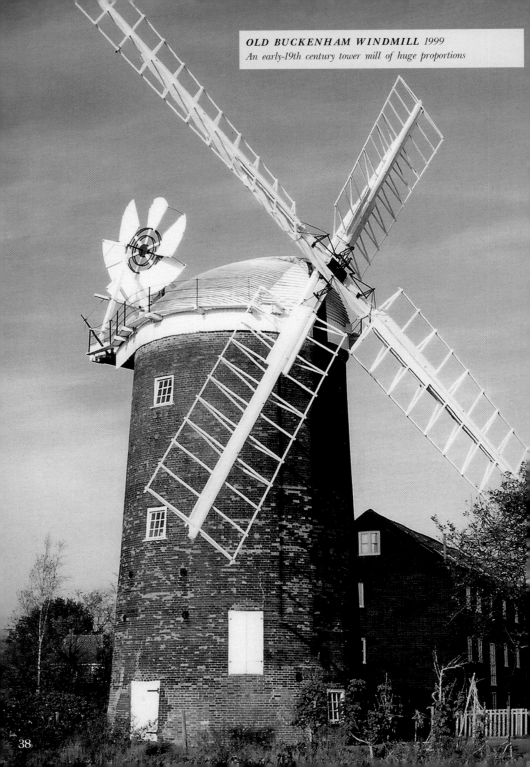

Garboldisham Mill TM 003805

*The last original **post mill** in Norfolk, Garboldisham Mill was known for many years as a spectacular derelict. It was saved from imminent collapse in 1972 by an enthusiastic new owner, Adrian Colman. Together with two friends, Philip Lennard and Philip Unwin, Adrian completely rebuilt the timber trestle with the mill body propped perilously above it.*

Between 1820 and 1837 three windmills, a post, a tower and a smock, stood on Garboldisham common. The surviving post mill, thought to have been built in the 1770s, is the oldest of the three. Its internal machinery was modernised around 1830 when the present iron gearing, which drives two pairs of 'underdrift' millstones in the head of the mill, was installed. Two of the original four sails were lost in a storm in 1906 and the mill finished its working life 11 years later using one pair of sails only. The mill body, or buck, is the longest in Norfolk at almost 22 feet (6.7 m). The buck contains three floors and is clad in white weatherboards, with a metal-covered roof. The oak trestle which supports the buck is housed in a circular brick roundhouse with a roof of tarred, felted boarding. The eight-bladed fantail, mounted above the rear ladder, turns the whole mill around to face the wind. Apart from its missing sails, the mill is now in first-class order (see p6) and flour is produced in the roundhouse using a modern milling machine.

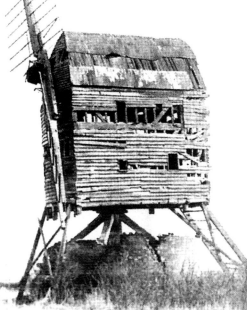

GARBOLDISHAM WINDMILL *Derelict, 1972*

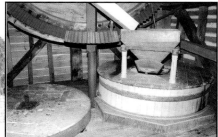

*The **BIN FLOOR** (above) and the **STONE FLOOR** (below), 1999*

Billingford Mill TM 167785

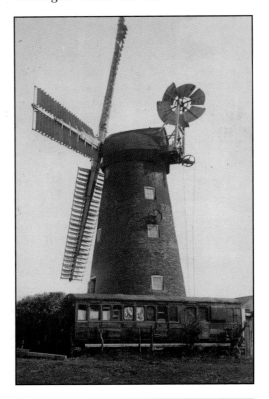

*An attractive brick **tower mill**, restored to a non-working condition in 1962 and brought into full working order in 1998. The mill has the distinction of being the last to work commercially in the county and was the first windmill to be acquired by the County Council for preservation.*

Billingford tower mill was built in 1859-60, at a cost of £1,300. It replaced a post mill which, rather inconsiderately, blew over with the miller, George Goddard still inside! Arthur Daines, Billingford's last miller, gave up using wind power in 1956 following damage to the two remaining sails although he continued working the mill until 1959, using auxiliary power. The mill was then purchased by Victor Valiant with a view to its preservation; he gave the mill to Norfolk County Council in 1962 on completion of the restoration work. A set of picturesque outbuildings, which included an old railway carriage, once surrounded the mill.

BILLINGFORD WINDMILL. The remains of the old post mill, October 1859 (below).
The new tower mill in working order, 1934 (above). Note the ancient railway carriage set up for use as a storage building

There are four wide double-shuttered sails of the patent type. The boat-shaped cap was tarred in the mill's latter working years but is now painted white. The unusually-shaped six-bladed fantail replaced one of a more traditional design in the 1930s. The tower has five storeys, the millstones being overdriven on the second floor. On a hurst frame on the ground floor of the tower is a separate pair of emery composition millstones. These were powered by an oil engine which had been installed in 1928.

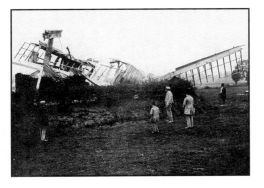

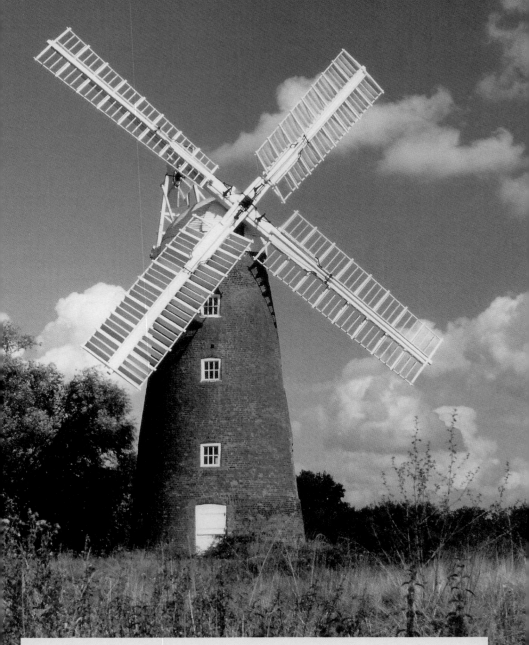

BILLINGFORD WINDMILL *1997*
A typical mid-19th century corn mill, now restored to working order and open to visitors

Drainage Mills of the River Ant

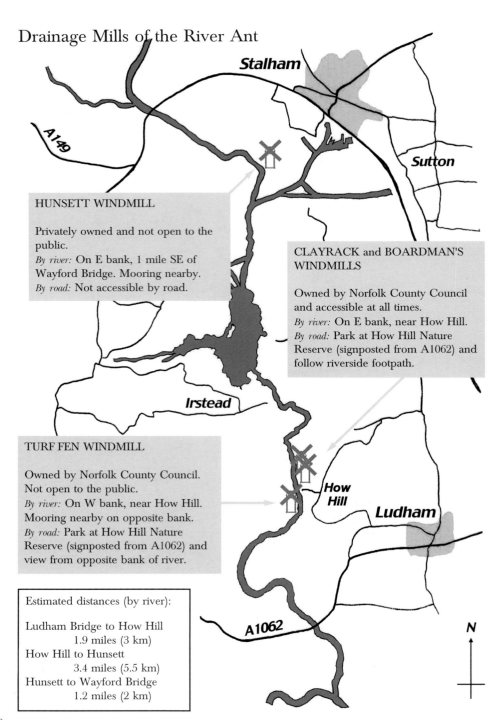

HUNSETT WINDMILL

Privately owned and not open to the public.
By river: On E bank, 1 mile SE of Wayford Bridge. Mooring nearby.
By road: Not accessible by road.

CLAYRACK and BOARDMAN'S WINDMILLS

Owned by Norfolk County Council and accessible at all times.
By river: On E bank, near How Hill.
By road: Park at How Hill Nature Reserve (signposted from A1062) and follow riverside footpath.

TURF FEN WINDMILL

Owned by Norfolk County Council. Not open to the public.
By river: On W bank, near How Hill. Mooring nearby on opposite bank.
By road: Park at How Hill Nature Reserve (signposted from A1062) and view from opposite bank of river.

Estimated distances (by river):

Ludham Bridge to How Hill
    1.9 miles (3 km)
How Hill to Hunsett
    3.4 miles (5.5 km)
Hunsett to Wayford Bridge
    1.2 miles (2 km)

42

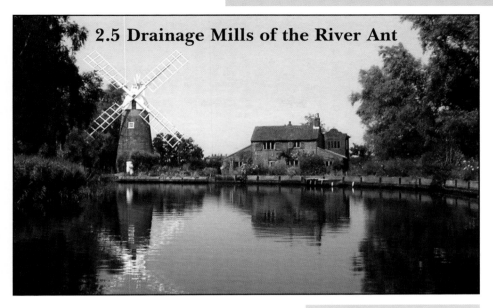

2.5 Drainage Mills of the River Ant

HUNSETT WINDMILL 1999

Hunsett Mill, Stalham TG 364239

*This brick **tower mill**, alongside its cottage in a picturesque corner of the Broads, is frequently seen on postcards although it has not functioned for many years. The name 'Hunsett' is thought to derive from an eel sett kept by a man named Hunn.*

Built in or around 1860, it stands on the site of a much older drainage mill. The tower is three storeys high but almost all the internal machinery except for the brake wheel has been removed. There is a small boat-shaped cap and a six-bladed fantail with distinctive red stripes. Unusually, the sails of this drainage mill drove twin scoop wheels placed on opposite sides of the tower. A large cast-iron belt pulley on the tower's exterior allowed the scoop wheels to be driven by an external auxiliary engine on days when there was not enough wind to turn the sails.

Clayrack Mill, How Hill TG 369194

*A diminutive **hollow-post mill** and one of the Broads' showpieces, Clayrack Mill was built in the mid- or late-19th century (at TG 367148) to drain a patch of Ranworth Marsh.*

Disused by 1905, Clayrack Mill gradually fell into a state of dereliction. In 1981 it was rescued, and was restored to working order in 1987-88 on its new site. The millwright responsible was Richard Seago who had previously rebuilt another hollow-post mill, Palmer's Mill, on a new site at Upton Marshes.

Clayrack Mill has an upright shaft driven by four small patent sails, each of which have only a single row of vanes. The sails are attached to the front of the tiny white-painted 'buck', which is balanced on the tarred wooden main post and is turned to face the wind by an eight-bladed fantail. Inside the buck, a pair of bevel gears operate the upright shaft which passes down through the hollow main post to the brick base of the mill. Here, within a tarred hoodway, a scoop wheel drains water from the adjoining marsh into the river.

Boardman's Mill, How Hill TG 370192

*Of a rare type known as a **skeleton mill**, Boardman's Mill resembles a four-sided smock mill without weatherboarding.*

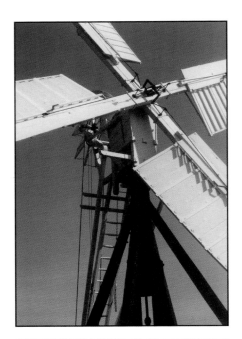

CLAYRACK WINDMILL 1999 (above)
BOARDMAN'S WINDMILL 2006 (below)

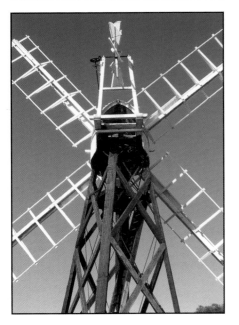

Although a scaled-down version of a tower mill, Boardman's Mill is nonetheless equipped with a miniature boat-shaped cap, six-bay patent sails and an eight-bladed fantail. The mill stands just under 30 feet (9.14m) high to the top of its cap. The four corner posts are supported on tarred brick piers and the cross bracing, which prevents the timber frame from distorting, can be clearly seen. A cast-iron spur pinion at the base of the mill's upright shaft drove an Appold turbine pump, which was fitted in place of the original scoop wheel in 1926. The turbine pump turns 7.2 times for every revolution of the sails. Boardman's Mill was built by millwright Dan England of Ludham in 1897 and operated until 1938 when it was severely damaged in a gale. After losing its cap, fantail and sails it was rescued and restored by the Norfolk Windmills Trust in 1981. Although able to turn itself to wind, it no longer works.

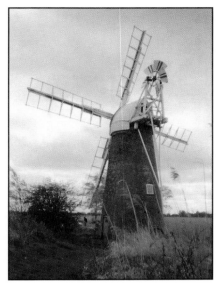

Turf Fen Mill, How Hill TG 369188

Similar in many respects to Hunsett Mill, Turf Fen **tower mill** *is one of only three such drainage mills known to have driven twin scoop wheels.*

The mill was built circa 1860 by the Stalham millwright William Rust, and remained in regular use until the 1940s. It stood derelict for many years until it was taken over by the Norfolk Windmills Trust in 1976. Assisted by Wymondham joiner Adrian Bond, millwright John Lawn restored Turf Fen Mill to a non-working condition between 1981 and 1986.

The characteristic boat-shaped cap, with its deep petticoat, is turned into wind by a six-bladed fantail, and runs on a shot curb. Inside the cap, mounted on the iron windshaft, is the fine head wheel of oak and elm, with its 57 applewood cogs. Iron gearing on the ground floor allowed either one or both scoop wheels to be driven, depending on the amount of wind available.

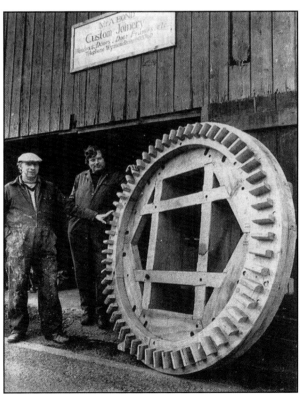

(above)
TURF FEN WINDMILL
with its red- and white-striped fantail, 1998

(large picture)
JOHN LAWN *(right) collects the new head wheel for Turf Fen Mill, made by* **ADRIAN BOND** *of Wymondham, in February 1985*

45

Drainage Mills of the River Thurne

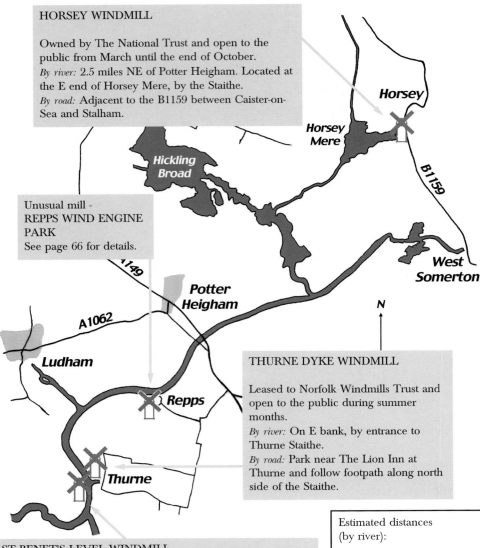

HORSEY WINDMILL

Owned by The National Trust and open to the public from March until the end of October.
By river: 2.5 miles NE of Potter Heigham. Located at the E end of Horsey Mere, by the Staithe.
By road: Adjacent to the B1159 between Caister-on-Sea and Stalham.

Unusual mill - REPPS WIND ENGINE PARK
See page 66 for details.

Hickling Broad

Horsey

Horsey Mere

B1159

West Somerton

1149

Potter Heigham

A1062

Ludham

Repps

N

THURNE DYKE WINDMILL

Leased to Norfolk Windmills Trust and open to the public during summer months.
By river: On E bank, by entrance to Thurne Staithe.
By road: Park near The Lion Inn at Thurne and follow footpath along north side of the Staithe.

Thurne

ST BENET'S LEVEL WINDMILL

Owned by Crown Estates and open to the public occasionally.
By river: Situated on W bank, 0.25 miles N of Thurne Mouth.
By road: From A1062, E of Ludham Bridge, turn into Hall Road. Continue S on concrete road and then follow footpath along riverbank.

Estimated distances (by river):

Thurne Staithe to Potter Heigham Bridge
2.8 miles (4.5 km)
Potter Heigham Bridge to Horsey Staithe
4.3 miles (7km)

2.6 Drainage Mills of the River Thurne

St Benet's Level Mill, Thurne TG 399156

*The most unusual feature of this **tower mill** is its ten-bladed fantail, one of only two examples left in the country.*

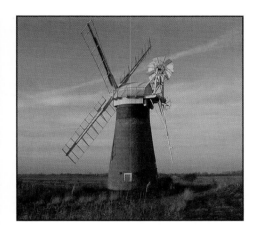

***ST BENET'S LEVEL WINDMILL** 2000*

This red brick drainage mill is owned by the Crown Estate. It was built in the 18th century and has since been heightened. The added brickwork, which is tarred, can be clearly seen. There are four long patent sails with nine double bays, and these drove an Appold turbine. The distinctive cap gallery and fantail reflect those of Sutton corn mill and represent the work of Daniel England, the Ludham millwright. Unusually, the mill was once fitted with an *annular* or circular sail, but this came to grief in a storm early in the 20th century. The mill was restored to a non-working condition in 1973-75 and again in 1989-90.

Thurne Dyke Mill TG 401159

*Thurne is a good example of a **tower mill** that has been heightened, or 'hained' as the Broadland millwrights termed it. The upper section of the tower was made cylindrical in order to re-use the existing cap and this has given the tower a marked 'waist'.*

This famous white-painted tower mill has stood guard over the entrance to Thurne Staithe since it was built in 1820 for the Commissioners of Drainage. The cap and sails were blown into the marsh when the mill was tailwinded in 1919. It was purchased for preservation in June 1949 by R.D. Morse (see p67) who carried out the restoration work with the help of millwright Albert England. It was later leased by the Norfolk Windmills Trust and was restored to working order in 2002 by millwright Vincent Pargeter. The eight-bladed fantail is decorated with red stripes, which were a feature of England's work. Iron gearing inside the tower drove a turbine pump which had ceased to be used by the end of World War II. Together with the restored St. Benet's Level Mill on the opposite bank of the river it forms an imposing sight in the flat landscape.

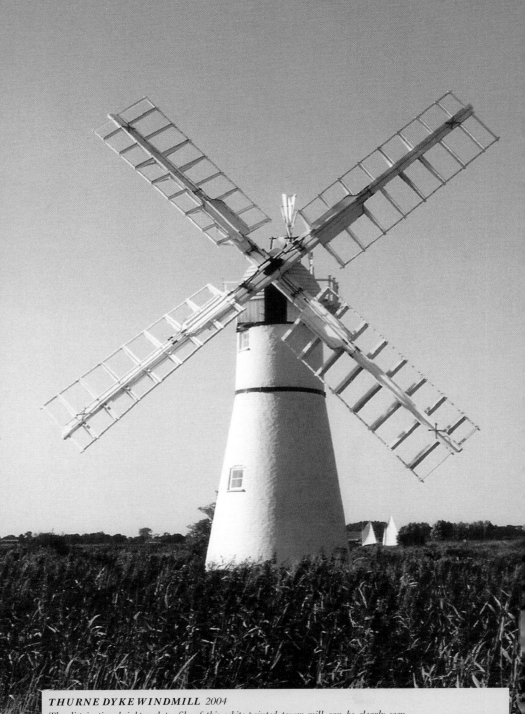

THURNE DYKE WINDMILL *2004*
The distinctive, heightened profile of this white-painted tower mill can be clearly seen

Horsey Mill TG 457221

*Horsey **tower mill** is one of the youngest drainage mills in the county, having been built in 1911-12 by England's of Ludham on the foundations of an 18th-century mill. Much of the internal gearing from the previous mill was re-used in the reconstruction.*

A well-known and substantial tower mill of four storeys, it has four patent sails and a large boat-shaped cap with a gallery and an eight-bladed fantail. The sails operated a turbine pump housed in the small weatherboarded structure attached to the tower. Twenty year-old Arthur Dove assisted with the construction of the mill and became the last man to operate it, having taken over as millman from his father in October 1918. A stationary steam engine supplemented the power of the wind for some time, and old photographs show a tall steam engine chimney standing close to the mill.

In July 1943 a lightning strike put the four sails out of action and the diesel pump, which had been installed in 1939 to assist the windmill, took over. In 1957, the diesel pump was replaced with an electric one. During the infamous floods of 1953, the mill became completely surrounded by sea water. Following a public appeal, Horsey Mill was restored in 1959-62 by Thomas Smithdale & Sons, millwrights of Acle.

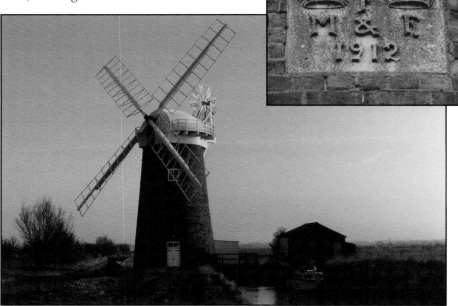

***HORSEY WINDMILL** and staithe, 1986. The inset photograph shows the datestone near the base of the mill commemorating its rebuilding in 1912*

Drainage Mills of the River Bure

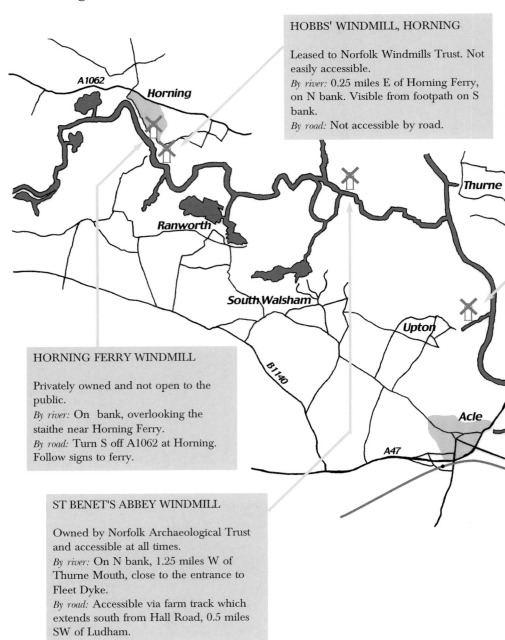

HOBBS' WINDMILL, HORNING

Leased to Norfolk Windmills Trust. Not easily accessible.
By river: 0.25 miles E of Horning Ferry, on N bank. Visible from footpath on S bank.
By road: Not accessible by road.

HORNING FERRY WINDMILL

Privately owned and not open to the public.
By river: On bank, overlooking the staithe near Horning Ferry.
By road: Turn S off A1062 at Horning. Follow signs to ferry.

ST BENET'S ABBEY WINDMILL

Owned by Norfolk Archaeological Trust and accessible at all times.
By river: On N bank, 1.25 miles W of Thurne Mouth, close to the entrance to Fleet Dyke.
By road: Accessible via farm track which extends south from Hall Road, 0.5 miles SW of Ludham.

ASHTREE FARM WINDMILL

Privately owned and leased to Norfolk
Windmills Trust. Not open to the public.
By river: On the S bank, 2 miles NE of
Great Yarmouth.
By road: Not accessible by road.

LMER'S WINDMILL, UPTON

vately owned. Accessible at all times.
river: At W end of Upton Dyke.
road: 1 mile NE of Upton. Park at
nic site and follow footpath to
oring.

STRACEY ARMS WINDMILL

Owned by Norfolk County Council and open
to the public during summer months.
By river: On S bank, 2.5 miles SE of Acle
Bridge.
By road: Adjacent to A47 between Norwich
and Great Yarmouth. Parking nearby.

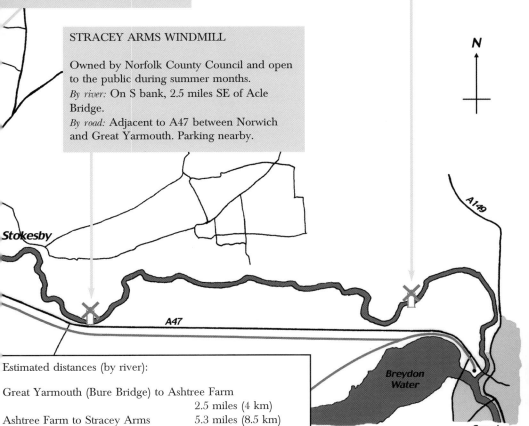

N

Stokesby

A149

A47

Breydon
Water

Great
Yarmouth

Estimated distances (by river):

Great Yarmouth (Bure Bridge) to Ashtree Farm

	2.5 miles (4 km)
Ashtree Farm to Stracey Arms	5.3 miles (8.5 km)
Stracey Arms to Upton Staithe	5.3 miles (8.5 km)
Upton Staithe to St Benet's Abbey	3.7 miles (6 km)
St Benet's Abbey to Horning	3.1 miles (5 km)

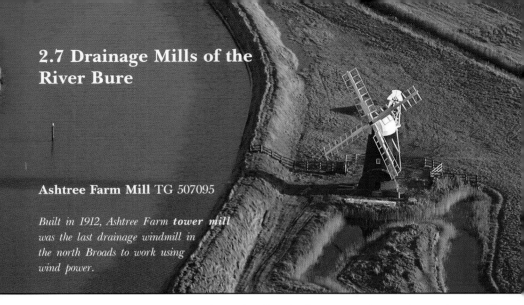

2.7 Drainage Mills of the River Bure

Ashtree Farm Mill TG 507095

*Built in 1912, Ashtree Farm **tower mill** was the last drainage windmill in the north Broads to work using wind power.*

A small mill of three storeys, it drained a detached area of Acle marshes and reputedly could lift eight tons of water every minute in a 15 m.p.h. wind. There are four patent sails, a boat-shaped cap and a six-bladed fantail. The sails drive a set of cast-iron machinery, some of which is second-hand and was fitted in place of the original wooden gear in the 1940s. The external scoop wheel is 16 feet (4.88 m) in diameter and 7 inches (18 cm) wide. The windmill was brought to a sudden halt by the storm of 31st January 1953, the night of the great East Coast flood when sea defences were breached and Yarmouth was flooded. For many years afterwards the structure stood derelict, its wooden cap roof gradually disintegrating. The mill's fortunes have recently taken a turn for the better, as it has been restored to turning order by Richard Seago as part of the 'Land of the Windmills' project. It was first necessary to level up the tower, which had developed a pronounced lean. A completely new cast-iron windshaft was also needed, as the original had broken during the storm.

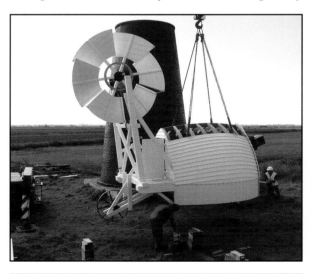

ASHTREE FARM WINDMILL *2006*
(top) The restored mill, behind its protective river bank
(bottom) A mobile crane lifts on the new cap and fantail

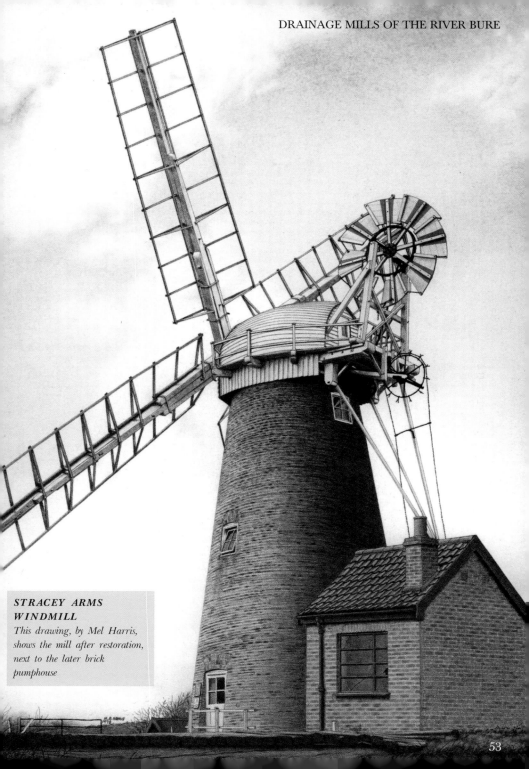

STRACEY ARMS
WINDMILL
This drawing, by Mel Harris,
shows the mill after restoration,
next to the later brick
pumphouse

Stracey Arms Mill, Tunstall TG 442090

*This sails of this brick **tower mill**, known as Arnup's Mill, are unusual in that they turn clockwise when viewed from the front.*

The present red brick tower mill, built in 1883, replaced an earlier structure which had been operated since 1831 by the Arnup family. Fred Mutton took over as millman in the 1940s and, although still in good order, the sails ceased to turn in 1946 when they were replaced by a 20 horse-power electric pump. A typical mill of the period, the cast-iron gearing inside is finely executed and drove an Appold turbine which replaced the original scoop wheel. The iron windshaft bears the date 1880 while the upright shaft carries the date 1883 as well as the millwright's name, "R BARNES GREAT YARMOUTH". When surveyed in 1959 the mill required extensive restoration as both its brickwork and woodwork had suffered damage through its use as a fortified post during World War II. The owner, Lady Stracey, conveyed the mill to Norfolk County Council as well as providing a generous grant for the restoration fund. Smithdale's, millwrights of Acle, commenced repair work on the mill in October 1960. A new cap gallery, two stocks, four patent sail frames, and an eight-bladed fantail were provided. Today, the mill again awaits extensive repair.

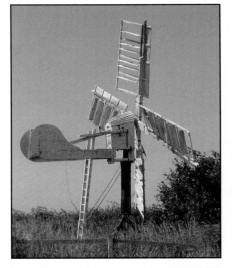

Palmer's Mill, Upton TG 403129

*The first restored **hollow-post mill** in Norfolk to pump water. It did so on 9th July 1980.*

Palmer's Mill is an intriguing, late-built example of an early style of drainage mill. It originally stood at Acle, near the present roundabout (at TG 404103). Built in the early-20th century, it had fallen into dereliction after ceasing work in the 1920s. The remains of the mill were rescued in 1976 and restored, at their present site, in 1977-80. The work was

PALMER'S WINDMILL, UPTON 2006
A diminutive hollow-post drainage mill

undertaken as a voluntary exercise by Richard Seago, who received a conservation award for the project.

The mill has a tiny, white-painted wooden buck supported by a tarred main post and trestle. There are four spring sails which span 21 feet 9 inches (6.63 m). These are fitted to the cranked cast-iron windshaft which, via a vertical crankshaft, operates a plunger pump set below ground level. The mill is steered into wind by twin tail vanes.

St Benet's Abbey Mill, Horning TG 380158

*The monastic site of St Benedict's or St Benet's Abbey contains the archaeological remains of a Benedictine Priory which was abandoned in 1545. The largest upstanding remnants of the buildings are the ruins of the Abbey gatehouse, around which a large brick **tower mill** was constructed circa 1740.*

One of the first tower mills to be built in the county, it started life as an industrial mill before being converted to a drainage mill, with a scoop wheel. Instead of milling corn, the windmill crushed locally-grown cole and rape seed for processing into oil. Nineteenth century photographs survive showing the primitive features of this remarkable structure. A wide access platform, or staging, around the tower was supported on top of the gatehouse walls and allowed the millman access to the tips of the four clockwise sails. By the mid-19th century, one pair of sails were of the hand-clothed *common* type, while the other pair had been replaced by a set of *spring sails* containing adjustable, spring-loaded vanes. The cap was an unusual conical shape - which was likely to have pre-dated the boat-shaped design - and was manually turned into wind by a braced tailpole. The windmill ceased work in 1863 when it was tailwinded and the sails were destroyed. Only the empty brick tower of the mill, standing 34 feet 5 inches (10.5 m) high, remains today.

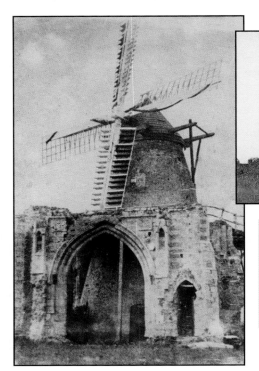

ST BENET'S ABBEY WINDMILL, HORNING

The surviving brick tower, shown above, appears rather out of place amidst the ruins of the Abbey gatehouse. The photograph on the left shows the mill in working order, and must date from around 1860

Hobbs' Mill, Horning TG 347163

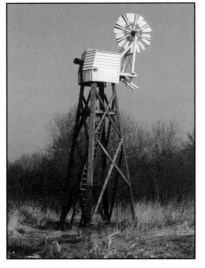

*Hobbs' Mill is one of only three **skeleton mills** to survive on the Broads and shares close similarities with the modified example at St Olaves.*

Built in the late-19th century, the mill ceased drainage work in the 1930s. By the 1970s it had become derelict, shorn of its cap, sails and fantail and leaning precariously due to a tree which had grown around its foundations. During the 1980s, Hobbs' Mill was partly restored using a grant from the nearby boatyard. Millwright John Lawn - assisted by builder Peter Sugden and volunteer David Alderton - undertook structural repairs and installed a new cap. The fantail had eight blades and there were four patent sails which drove a scoop wheel at the base of the tower.

(above) **HOBBS' WINDMILL, HORNING** *1990*
(below) **HORNING FERRY WINDMILL** *in working order, c 1900*

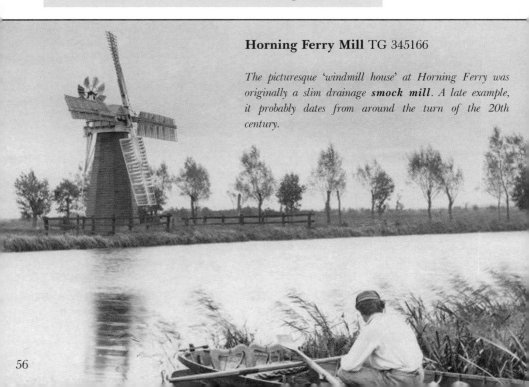

Horning Ferry Mill TG 345166

*The picturesque 'windmill house' at Horning Ferry was originally a slim drainage **smock mill**. A late example, it probably dates from around the turn of the 20th century.*

During the process of conversion to a holiday home the mill's appearance has been considerably altered, and the ground floor extended to provide additional living space. This process has given the tower a 'flared' profile. Old photographs show the windmill in its working days, its straight-sided tower covered with tarred weatherboarding. The boat-shaped cap was painted white and there were four patent sails. Today, the entire structure is white and the sails have been replaced with dummy ones. Fortunately, several original features survive, including the cap gallery and an unusual seven-bladed fantail.

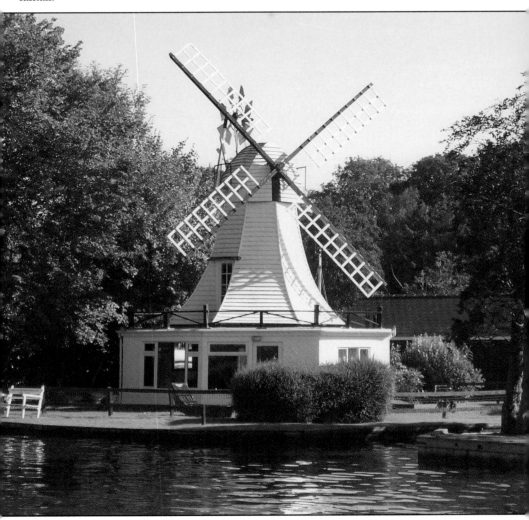

HORNING FERRY WINDMILL *converted to living accommodation, 2007. The main elements of the original mill are still in place*

Drainage Mills of the River Yare & River Waveney

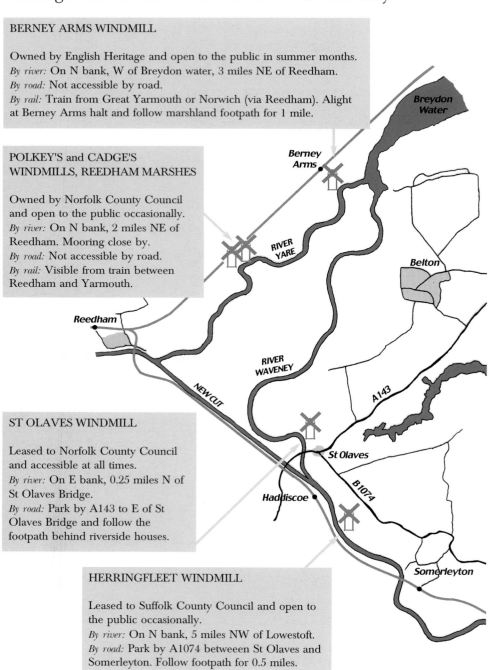

BERNEY ARMS WINDMILL

Owned by English Heritage and open to the public in summer months.
By river: On N bank, W of Breydon water, 3 miles NE of Reedham.
By road: Not accessible by road.
By rail: Train from Great Yarmouth or Norwich (via Reedham). Alight at Berney Arms halt and follow marshland footpath for 1 mile.

POLKEY'S and CADGE'S WINDMILLS, REEDHAM MARSHES

Owned by Norfolk County Council and open to the public occasionally.
By river: On N bank, 2 miles NE of Reedham. Mooring close by.
By road: Not accessible by road.
By rail: Visible from train between Reedham and Yarmouth.

ST OLAVES WINDMILL

Leased to Norfolk County Council and accessible at all times.
By river: On E bank, 0.25 miles N of St Olaves Bridge.
By road: Park by A143 to E of St Olaves Bridge and follow the footpath behind riverside houses.

HERRINGFLEET WINDMILL

Leased to Suffolk County Council and open to the public occasionally.
By river: On N bank, 5 miles NW of Lowestoft.
By road: Park by A1074 betweeen St Olaves and Somerleyton. Follow footpath for 0.5 miles.

Breydon Water

Berney Arms

RIVER YARE

Belton

Reedham

RIVER WAVENEY

NEW CUT

A143

St Olaves

B1074

Haddiscoe

Somerleyton

2.8
Drainage
Mills of the
River Yare

Estimated distances (by river):	
Reedham boatyard to Seven Mile House	2.8 miles (4.5 km)
Seven Mile House to Berney Arms	1.9 miles (3 km)
Berney Arms to Bure Bridge, Great Yarmouth	4.3 miles (7 km)
Bure Bridge, Great Yarmouth to St Olaves	9 miles (14.5 km)
St Olaves to Herringfleet	1.6 miles (2.5 km)
Herringfleet to Mutford Bridge, Lowestoft	6.2 miles (10 km)

Polkey's Mill (TG 444034) and **Cadge's Mill** (TG 446035) and the Reedham Steam Engine House are situated at **Seven Mile House** by the River Yare on **Reedham Marshes**.

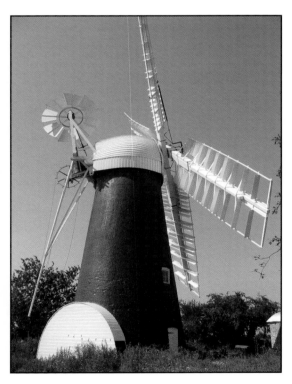

This group of buildings illustrates the four forms of power which have been used, over the years, to drain the marshes. They demonstrate how wind power could be used in conjunction with steam or diesel power, all of which were eventually superseded by electricity.

POLKEY'S WINDMILL, REEDHAM MARSHES 2006
Restored to working order. The white-painted woodwork contrasts sharply with the tarred brick tower

An old, three-storey tower mill, Polkey's Mill displays many intriguing features including three different phases of brickwork which suggest it has been heightened twice. The main timbers of the upper two floors appear to have come from an earlier drainage mill on the site, a timber-towered smock mill. The four large patent sails span 70 feet (21.34 m) and, unusually, rotate clockwise when viewed from the front. The elegant boat-shaped cap has an eight-bladed fantail. Inside, the gearing is entirely of cast iron, with wooden cogs in the head wheel and pit wheels. The sails drive a large scoop wheel within a white-painted timber hoodway adjacent to the tower. The scoop wheel turns 8.25 times for every ten revolutions of the sails.

Polkey's Mill was built some time in the 19th century and in its heyday could pump 40 tons of water every minute in a good wind. The adjacent steam pump was installed in the 1880s but the windmill worked in partnership with the fossil-fuelled machinery until the 1940s. By the 1950s the mill had lost its roof and some of the internal machinery had been removed for scrap. Following protection work in the 1970s, Polkey's Mill was skilfully restored to full working order by Vincent Pargeter and his team between 2002 and 2005.

Cadge's Mill, also known as Batchie's and Stimpson's Mill, is a large, powerful tower mill. It was probably built circa 1870 by Thomas Smithdale of Norwich, whose name appears on the cast-iron windshaft.

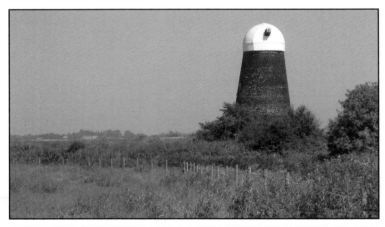

CADGE'S WINDMILL, REEDHAM MARSHES with its new cap, 2006

Cadge's Mill differs from Polkey's in that the four patent sails rotated anti- clockwise. The scoop wheel which they drove is located inside the tower and, at 20 feet (6.1 m) in diameter by 12 inches (0.3 m) wide, was a relatively large example. The new boat-shaped cap, which replicates the very rounded original, was lifted into place early in 2006. Unusual features of the brick tower include two heating stoves on the ground floor. These served to keep the marshman warm on cold winter evenings, and also helped to prevent the internal scoop wheel from freezing solid in its culvert.

The mill was at the centre of a court case in September 1932, when farmer Frederick Key of Mundham refused to pay £8 in drainage rates to mill owner Arthur Stimpson. Key's defence was that drainage had not been carried out, or at least had been done so negligently as to be of no value! In 1941, the four sails were removed by Reggie Hewitt for use at another mill, and later still all the machinery below the cap was removed. Vincent Pargeter has restored the curb, windshaft and cap, although there are no sails or fantail at present and the missing machinery has not been replaced.

Berney Arms Mill TG 465049

*This superb **tower mill** is thought to have been built solely for cement grinding by Edmund Stolworthy of Great Yarmouth in 1865 for the Berney Family, and later converted to become the tallest drainage mill in Broadland. With a span of 85 feet (25.9 m), the mill's sails are the longest on any windmill in the UK.*

As mill authority Rex Wailes explained, *"the chalky mud dredged from the river was burned to produce cement clinker; this was ground in the mill by three pairs of 4' 6" (1.37 m) diameter Peak stones situated on the second floor. At the same time the steam cement works at Burgh Castle used to send clinker by wherry to be ground at the mill."* The works closed in 1880 and by 1883 the mill had been converted for drainage use. After ceasing work in 1949 it was taken into the care of the Ministry of Works who commissioned a thorough

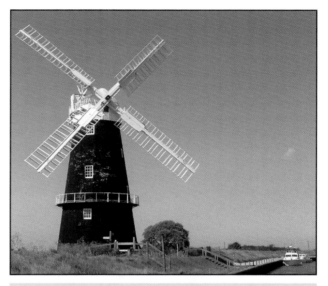

BERNEY ARMS WINDMILL, *recently restored, 2007*

restoration between 1965 and 1967. The mill has been extensively restored during the 21st century; in November 2002 the boat-shaped cap was removed by crane and transported to Leicestershire where it was fully repaired. It was replaced in May 2003 and the restoration was completed in 2007.

The windmill stands 70 feet 6 inches (21.56 m) tall over the cap with a tarred tower of seven storeys. There is an iron reefing stage at third-floor level. The elegant boat-shaped cap, with its gently curving ridge, has an iron-railed gallery and is turned into wind by an eight-bladed fantail. A notable feature, as seen on many Broadland mills, is the striking chain guide pole which extends down from the rear of the cap and prevents the chain from swinging about in gusty weather. The iron upright shaft and wallower are driven by a wooden clasp-arm brake wheel of oak, 9 feet 10 inches (3 m) in diameter, surrounded by a brake of poplar. On the ground floor, two cast-iron mitre gears (equal size bevels) transmit power to a huge scoop wheel located some distance from the tower. The wheel is 26 feet 6 inches (4.05 m) in diameter and turns seven times for every 20 revolutions of the sails, lifting water to a height of 8 feet (2.44 m).

2.9 Drainage Mills of the River Waveney

St Olaves Mill TM 457997

*An earlier smock mill on this site, which was very similar to the surviving mill at Herringfleet, was demolished in 1898. It was succeeded by the present four-sided timber drainage mill. Built in 1910 by Dan England of Ludham, this was known as 'Priory Mill'. It was originally constructed as an open-framed **skeleton mill** - similar to Hobbs' mill at Horning - and later, in 1928, gained its cladding of horizontal weatherboards.*

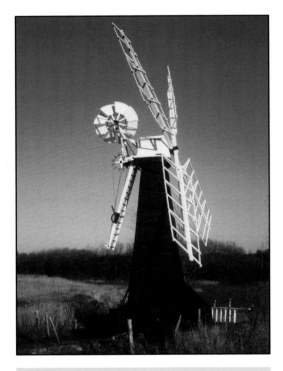

ST OLAVES WINDMILL
Following the first restoration of the 1980s

The mill has a tiny, straight-sided cap with an eight-bladed fantail. Its four patent sails drive an internal scoop wheel. A narrow ladder descends from the rear of the cap, giving access for repairs and maintenance. St Olaves Mill ceased work in 1957 when it was superseded by an electric pump. It was restored to working order between December 1974 and March 1981, and has recently been extensively overhauled. Sadly, the mill was severely damaged in the storms of January 2007. Until border changes occurred in 1974, the mill stood in Suffolk.

Herringfleet Mill TM 465976

*Although strictly a Suffolk mill, Herringfleet **smock mill** is an important element of the East Anglian scene, being the only full-sized drainage smock mill on the Broads to survive in a complete condition. An interesting feature of the mill is the ground-floor fireplace which helped the marshman keep warm on cold winter nights.*

Herringfleet Mill was probably built by James Barnes of Reedham circa 1830, and its survival is largely to the credit of the Somerleyton Estate who kept it working as long as was economically possible. The last estate marshman was Charlie Howlett, a fine local character whose distinctive regional dialect was fortunately recorded for posterity

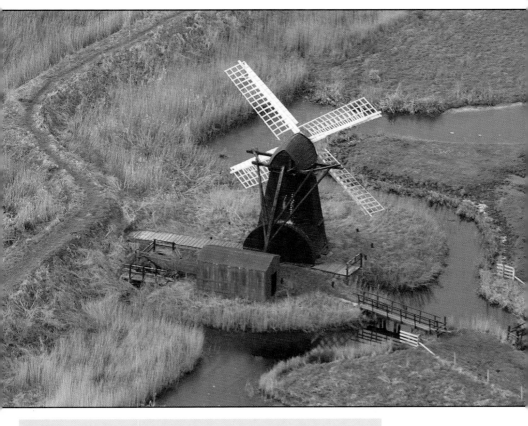

HERRINGFLEET WINDMILL 2006
The mill drains the marshland on the left into the meandering river

by local journalists and film-makers. Charlie operated the mill from 1923 until the scoop wheel sustained damage in 1955.

The octagonal timber-framed tower of the mill, clad in tarred weatherboarding, stands on a low brick base. From the boat-shaped cap, a braced tailpole extends downwards, and a chain winch fitted at its end enables the cap to be hauled around to face the wind. The four common sails rotate anti-clockwise and are spread with sheets of ochre-coloured canvas to catch the wind. The sails operate an externally-placed scoop wheel 9 inches (22.9 cm) wide and 16 feet (4.88 m) in diameter. The head wheel, wallower and upright shaft are of timber while the pit gears are of cast iron, with wooden cogs in the pit wheel. With the sails turning at a speed of 15 r.p.m., the mill lifts water at an estimated rate of 2000 gallons (9000 litres) every minute. The mill is regularly operated on public open days by volunteers from the Suffolk Mills Group.

2.10 Unusual Mills

Union Mills, Burnham Overy TF 842426 (see map p28)

Only a handful of combined wind- and watermills were constructed in Britain, and two of these stand in Norfolk. The country's surviving examples differ significantly in design, and most of them enjoyed limited success in their working lives, perhaps because it was difficult to find locations that met the needs of both types of mill. Windmills work best in raised, unobstructed landscapes whereas watermills require a reliable, year-round water supply - factors which can be mutually exclusive.

Thomas Beeston built a six-storey tower mill adjoining the existing watermill on the River Burn in 1814, a date inscribed on the mill's exterior. The windmill could run three pairs of millstones, providing additional capacity to the watermill which operated four pairs. Flour dressing machinery inside the watermill could also be operated by wind power through a system of shafts and gears. A sale notice from 1825 boasted that the four sails were fitted with an unusual feature - vanes made of copper. By 1893 the windmill's working life had ceased and its contents were offered for auction. The windmill's wide timber reefing stage and ogee cap with gallery have been reconstructed during recent work to convert the tower into a residence. The watermill still contains much of its original machinery, including an iron waterwheel which turns for demonstration.

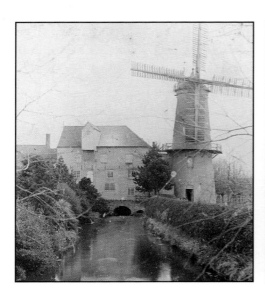 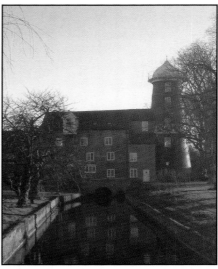

BURNHAM OVERY COMBINED MILL *in working order, c1900 (left) and converted to a residence, with replica cap and reefing stage, 2007 (right)*

Little Cressingham combined wind- and watermill TF 870002 (see map p36)

In 1780 local maps showed only a watermill at this site. It is thought that the present brick tower mill was built in 1821. The wooden machinery from a nearby smock mill may well have been re-used in the present tower mill because the craftsmanship of the wind-driven gearing contrasts sharply with the cast-iron machinery that is water driven. Miller Samuel Goddard and his wife Elizabeth were suffocated in the mill house on Christmas night 1890 when they took a bucketful of hot coals up to their bedroom to keep themselves warm. Wind power ceased to be used following a tailwinding in 1916. The Freestone family came to Cressingham in 1907 and, when milling by wind was discontinued, a Blackstone oil engine was coupled up to the

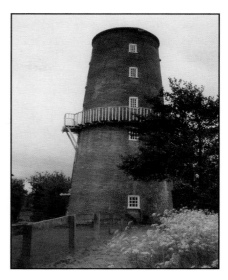

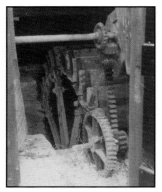

LITTLE CRESSINGHAM COMBINED MILL 1994 (above).
The principal waterwheel and sluice gears, 1986 (left)

water-driven stones to help out in dry periods. Two years later a Tattershall Roller Mill was installed and this was used intermittently until 1952 when the mill closed down. The mill was conveyed to the Norfolk Windmills Trust in 1981, when restoration commenced.

The boat-shaped cap with its gallery and windshaft were removed in the 1940s when a flat roof was placed over the tower. This roof, although never completed, protected much of the machinery until restoration of the mill began. The tall tower has six storeys with a wooden reefing stage at third-floor level. This was the windmill's meal floor and contains the lower section of the upright shaft which is elegantly stop-chamfered. A wooden clasp-arm spur wheel drove a pair of peak and a pair of French stones on the floor above. Another pair of each type of millstone remain on the first floor; these were driven by an iron breast-shot waterwheel, 12 feet (3.66 m) in diameter and 6 feet (1.83 m) wide. An oat crusher on the second floor was also water-powered. Beside the mill is a gothic-style pumphouse, built in the early-19th century and containing a separate, smaller waterwheel. This operated a Bramah pump which raised water up to the nearby Clermont House. During the 1930s, two hydraulic rams were installed to improve the system.

Morse's Wind Engine Park, Repps
TG 413162 (see map p46)

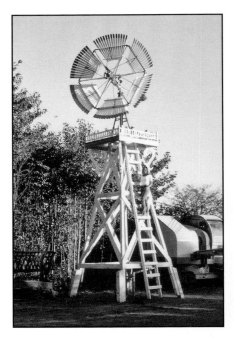

*Over five decades, Sussex native Bob Morse created a fascinating and unique open-air museum of **wind engines** at a site close to the River Thurne at Repps.*

Mr Morse, who passed away in January 2007, collected several interesting and unusual examples of wind engines from different parts of the UK and abroad. Many of these, such as the diminutive four-bladed windpump from Iwade in Kent (below right), have been rescued from a derelict state and painstakingly rebuilt.

Put simply, a wind engine is a mechanism for harnessing the power of the wind to drive pumps or other machinery. More particularly, it is a windmill which has been designed with mass-production in mind. Although they continue to be produced in small numbers today, the heyday of the wind engine was the period 1880-1930.

One of the most beautiful exhibits is a timber-framed 'Halladay' wind engine from North America with a set of self-regulating red and white blades that echo the form of a flower (above right).

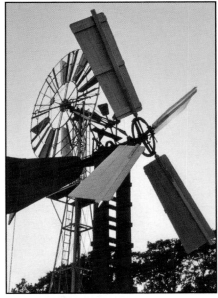

Another imported example is the modern 'Southern Cross' from New South Wales, Australia, with its three-sided metal tower. An easily recognisable feature of this wind engine is its annular sail which consists of a set of angled blades arranged in a circular formation. Although this type of sail is characteristic of wind engines across the globe, the first successful example was developed by an Essex miller, Henry Chopping, in the mid-19th century.

*(top) The **Halladay wind engine**.*
*(above) The **Iwade pump** with the **Minsmere wind engine** behind it*

66

A fine example of a wind engine with a fantail and an adjustable annular sail has been recovered from Minsmere Level nature reserve near Leiston on the Suffolk coast. Built in the 19th century by the celebrated engineer, John Wallis Titt of Warminster, Wiltshire, it is one of only two restored examples of its type in Britain.

At the centre of the site, a full-size scoop wheel from Whitlingham near Norwich has been set up within a fishpond to scoop water for demonstration. Visitors are offered a chance to see this dramatic piece of machinery in action.

A very fine stationary steam engine has been set up to drive an Appold turbine pump (see page 11). The engine, built by Holmes of Prospect Place, Norwich, is the only restored example of its kind.

The park's owners aim to ensure the long-term conservation of Mr Morse's collection, at the same time providing an unrivalled educational resource. The park offers a membership scheme which includes a twice-yearly publication, *The Morse Messenger*.

MORSE'S WIND ENGINE PARK *2004*
(below) A general view of the park during a visit from a group of enthusiasts. (right) The late Mr R D Morse

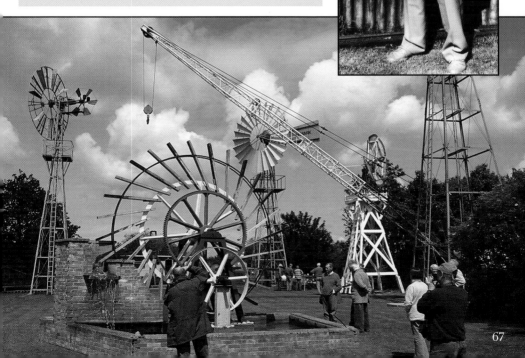

PART 3: PRESENT AND FUTURE

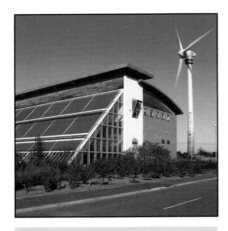

3.1 Generating electricity by wind power in Norfolk

*The tradition of using wind power in Norfolk is being continued by modern engineers. Wind-powered electricity generators, known as **wind turbines**, are part of the country's growing portfolio of renewable energy sources. The use of wind power reduces the amount of fossil fuels consumed in our quest for energy, and also limits the amount of carbon dioxide and other greenhouse gases released into the atmosphere.*

A modern wind turbine is not unlike a traditional windmill in design, as its three principal components are similar to those of a tower mill. Its own tower - nowadays of hollow steel construction - is proportionately much taller and slimmer than that of a traditional tower mill. On top, a streamlined cap, known as the *nacelle*, rotates through 360° to allow the sails, or blades, to face the oncoming wind. The nacelle is winded automatically by two powerful electric motors which are activated by a

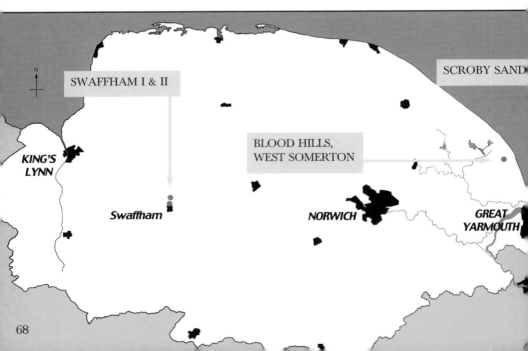

large weathervane, or direction indicator, protruding from the top. Most wind turbines have three fibreglass *blades*, instead of the traditional four sails, for reasons

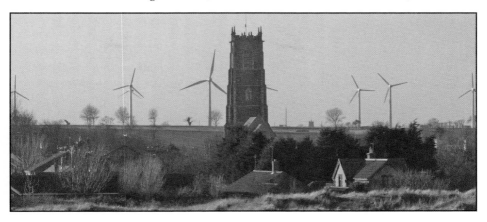

BLOOD HILLS WIND FARM, WEST SOMERTON 1999. *Some of the original Vestas turbines with the new, larger Ecotricity turbine in the centre*

of aerodynamic efficiency. In common with the traditional windmill, all of Norfolk's wind turbines are of the downwind type, meaning that the wind strikes the front surface of the blades rather than the rear.

Blood Hills Wind Farm, West Somerton
TG 477190

A group of ten wind turbines were commissioned at Blood Hills, near the east coast, in 1992. Each machine has an output of 225 kilowatts, giving a combined total of 2.25 megawatts; rather a low capacity in today's terms. The group are operated by E:ON-UK and the turbines were designed by Vestas.

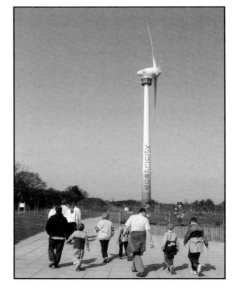

A pair of turbines at Swaffham

'SWAFFHAM I' WIND TURBINE

In 1999, the town of Swaffham in west Norfolk gained its own turbine. This is a much larger example that can generate 1.5 megawatts of power by itself - enough to supply the energy needs of 3,000 people, or more than one third of the whole town. 'Swaffham

I' was the first of a new generation of direct drive, variable speed turbines to be constructed in the UK and stands 219 feet 9 inches (67 m) high, with blades 101 feet 8 inches (31 m) in length. Part of the success of this turbine has been its relationship with local residents and tourists to the region, as it forms part of the Ecotech Centre, a state-of-the-art museum providing information about modern wind power and renewable energy sources. The highlight of a visit to the Centre is a chance to climb 300 steps inside the turbine to a viewing gallery 213 feet (65 m) above the ground - the only one of its kind in the UK. This commands fine views of the surrounding countryside as well as providing a rare, close-up view of the enormous turbine blades as they sweep past.

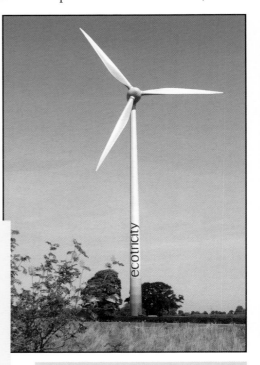

Vital statistics: Swaffham I, Ecotech Centre	
Installed	1999
Turbines	1
Capacity	1.5 MW
Generation (kWh)	3.5 million
Equivalent homes	1100
Hub height	67 m
Rotor diameter	66 m
Carbon dioxide savings	3161 tonnes
Sulphur dioxide savings	37 tonnes
Nitrogen oxide savings	11 tonnes

'SWAFFHAM II' WIND TURBINE,
built by public demand in 2003

The popularity of Swaffham's first turbine resulted in the construction of a second one in July 2003. Together, the pair supply 75% of the town's home electricity requirements. At the time of its completion, 'Swaffham II' was the UK's tallest onshore turbine, at 279 feet (85 m) high. Its enormous blades are 108 feet (33 m) long.

A big brother for West Somerton

The success of the Blood Hills site encouraged Ecotricity to construct a large machine here in July 2000 - an identical model to Swaffham I. The turbine took four days to construct. It provides 5% of Great Yarmouth's domestic electricity requirements - a staggering 4,500,000 units of pollution-free, 'green' electricity each year, benefiting over 4,000 local people.

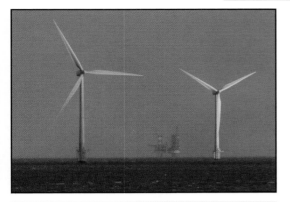

SCROBY SANDS OFFSHORE TURBINES

Scroby Sands offshore turbines
TG 565118

Part of the region's large offshore wind resource has also been tapped by the pioneering Scroby Sands Project. In 2004, a group of 30 colossal turbines were erected 2.5 km from the coast of Great Yarmouth and Caister-on-Sea, at a cost of £75 million.

Each of these giant machines generates 2 megawatts, providing a combined total for the wind farm of 60 megawatts - enough electricity to supply approximately 41,000 homes and save 75,000 tonnes of carbon dioxide every year.

EPILOGUE: 'Green' electricity from the Broadland drainage mills?

The use of wind as an energy resource may well come full circle if an innovative use of the Broadland drainage mills proves to be viable. Experts in the region have proposed a scheme to restore some of the remaining derelict drainage mills and use them to generate electricity for the National Grid. A report entitled *The possibility of converting former wind-pumps to produce electricity with computer control: a feasibility study* was jointly produced by two trustees of the Norfolk Windmills Trust and two scientists from Loughborough University's CREST Laboratory. The scheme proposes to install self-contained generating equipment inside the windpumps, at the same time restoring their exteriors to an authentic appearance with working caps, fantails and sails (right). The aim of the scheme is to increase the number of restored and operable mills on the Broads, thereby enhancing the visual impact of the area while making a useful contribution to Norfolk's energy needs.

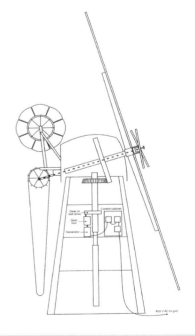

DESIGN FOR ELECTRICITY-GENERATING DRAINAGE MILL

71

Further information

Several books have been written about Norfolk, its corn and drainage mills, and English windmills in general. Although most of them are now out of print, the information they contain remains valuable. The following selection are highly recommended:

Apling, H. 1984. *Norfolk Corn Windmills*. The Norfolk Windmills Trust.
Detailed study of the county's surviving industrial windmills, with historical photographs.
Bowskill, D. 1999. *The Norfolk Broads and Fens*. OPUS Publishing.
Useful introduction to the county's navigable waterways from a boating perspective.
Hutchinson, S. 2000-07. *Berney Arms / Burgh Castle / Reedham Remembered and The Halvergate Fleet / The Haddiscoe Island - Past and Present*. S & P Hutchinson.
Five historical studies written from a family history perspective, containing fascinating insights into life and work in Broadland at around the turn of the 20th century.
Malster, R. *The Broads*. Phillimore.
A detailed historical study describing many aspects of Broadland life and lore.
Scott, M. 1977. *The Restoration of Windmills and Windpumps in Norfolk*. The N.W.T.
The story behind the movement to preserve Norfolk's unique windmill heritage.
Smith, A. C. 1982. *Corn Windmills in Norfolk*. Stevenage Museum Publications.
Location information for all visible corn windmill remains within the county.
Smith A. C. 1989. *Drainage Windmills of the Norfolk Marshes*. Arthur Smith Publications.
Location information for all visible drainage windmill remains within the county.
Wailes, R. 1957. *The English Windmill*. Routledge and Kegan Paul.
An unrivalled reference work covering the subject as a whole.
Watts, M. 2006. *Windmills* and *Watermills*. Shire Publications.
Clear, concise and reliable introductions to the variety of mills that survive in the UK.
Williamson, T. 1997. *The Norfolk Broads: A Landscape History*. Manchester University Press.
A geographical and archaeological study, with a detailed chapter on the drainage windmills.

Information about Norfolk mills is also available online. The most useful websites are:

Norfolk Mills	www.norfolkmills.co.uk
The Norfolk Windmills Trust	www.norfolkwindmills.co.uk
Windmill World	www.windmillworld.com
The Mills Archive	www.millsarchivetrust.org
S.P.A.B. Mills Section	www.spab.org.uk/mills
Ecotricity wind turbines	www.ecotricity.co.uk
E:ON-UK wind turbines	www.eon-uk.com

A note to visitors
Many of the mills featured in this book are open regularly during the summer months. For up-to-date opening times, look out for individual advertising leaflets, available from Tourist Information Centres and local attractions. All of the mills are visible from public rights of way, but most are, nevertheless, private property. During off-peak periods, please respect owners' privacy and do not trespass on the mill properties.

More details of the mills featured in this book, together with information for visitors, are available at **www.bonwick.co.uk**.

Index of drainage and corn windmills

Numbers shown in *italics* refer to illustrations.

Index of people